My Breast Cancer Adventure

OR WHAT CAN HAPPEN FOLLOWING A BREAST CANCER DIAGNOSIS

Plus Stories From Other Warriors

EMMA SCATTERGOOD

To my mum.

You were always there when I needed you.

CONTENTS

PART TWO – THEIR STORIES

PREFACE

The Breast Cancer Warrior

—⟨≫⟩—

HERE'S A LITTLE SOMETHING TO mull over. Something you've probably never consciously thought about. At this precise moment, there is someone out there, mentally preparing to have one or both of her breasts amputated. And there is someone, currently draining bloody fluid from a plastic tube that painfully protrudes from a hole in her torso. It doesn't stop there. At this exact moment and there are literally millions of women, all over the world, battling lymphoedema, treating weeping radiation burns, suffering debilitating nerve damage, vomiting from the side-effects of chemotherapy, hearing they may never have children, losing nails, fighting infections, going bald. All of these somebodies who I term breast cancer warriors will be combating exhaustion. Some will be learning their cancer has spread to their bones, their eye, their brain. Many will be dying.

Every time she feels an ache, the slightest pain, there is someone out there, terrified their cancer has returned, spread, metastasised. If she has withstood, conquered, survived her initial treatment, this someone may now be on an indefinite tablet that bleeds her body of essential hormones or a pill that causes appalling fatigue or diarrhoea. She may even now, be tethered to a hospital for the rest of her life. Having to return every few weeks for critical infusions.

These someones somewhere, some of whom I have met, are the warriors who are dealing with situations that most, going about their everyday lives, are not conscious of. Never even think about.

This book aims to bring awareness to how breast cancer can be diagnosed and what can happen once it has. It's mainly my story, my adventure, and it's not overly unusual, but it is the story of how I went from the ranks of the oblivious to a battler on the front line and it also includes accounts from some pretty incredible ladies, all of whom have had to face and fight this awful disease. I call it an adventure because that is what I am, an adventurer, and that is what it was—an undertaking involving danger and unknown risks. And it was written to not only offer guidance and support to fellow suffers—comfort through unity, but also, hopefully, to provide comprehension to the unaware.

PART ONE

My Story

CHAPTER

1

A Dimple on my Breast

———⁓———

IF YOU'RE AN AUSTRALIAN FEMALE aged thirty or over, then no doubt you have heard of Jane McGrath. She's the face of pink cricket. Her image splashed over your tv screen during the first cricket test of the Australian new year. The gorgeous gregarious English lass who had it all. Famous talented husband Glen, two beautiful boisterous young kids, jet setting lifestyle, elegance plus a charismatic bubbly personality. Then, at only 42, tragically young, lost it all to breast cancer. Well, it's Jane I must thank for kick-starting my breast cancer adventure. For creating a niggle that motivated me enough to stop procrastinating and provoked me into revisiting a doctor. It was only through recalling a documentary on Jane, made some years after her death, remembering fascinating footage of her explaining how she discovered her cancer, that eventually coerced me into picking up my phone and making an appointment. In the documentary, Jane talks about how she had taken a shower and afterwards, standing naked in front of the mirror, had noticed that something didn't look quite right with one of her breasts. Laughing, she then tells how, still naked, she asked her husband Glen for his advice and his unhelpful distraction with her damp bare breasts. It was a captivating documentary, not the least because Jane, despite her ongoing serious battle with breast cancer, could still laugh. It was an interview that fortunately, I couldn't forget.

In late September, maybe early October 2021, also standing damp and naked in front of a mirror, I thought that maybe, one of my breasts looked slightly different than usual. That the left one had a bit of a dimple to it or a flat plane. It was barely discernible, and unlike Jane, I wasn't overly concerned. For years, at least the past two decades, my breasts had seen me a regular visitor to both the doctor and the radiologist. Diagnosed with lumpy breast disease in my thirties, I was never without a few lumps in both breasts necessitating regular mammograms, ultrasounds, and the odd biopsy. It was common for me to be told by sonographers how lovely and 'dense' my breast tissue was. 'The breasts of a 20-year-old'. Having lumps in my breasts had become so common, so normal that although this time the breast did look slightly different, I had never had a dimple before; it didn't worry me enough to do anything about it. To cement this, in the back of my mind, I was remembering that just over 12 months ago, I had visited a breast and endocrine specialist who had reassured me that, according to a recent mammogram, all my breast lumps and bumps were perfectly normal.

The thing about a beautiful, funny, memorable lady telling a story about how she discovered her breast cancer after a shower, then every day looking at your own breasts after a shower, knowing things don't look quite the same as usual, is that eventually, uncertainty steps in and the guilt builds. Guilt that, despite the hassle of Covid, I should make another appointment to have my breasts checked yet again. Guilt that it's just laziness that's stopping me. Guilt that even though I don't think anything is wrong, maybe, just maybe, this time there is. It takes approximately nine weeks for the self-reproach to build enough for me to eventually pick up a phone to make an appointment to visit a doctor and even then, the appointment is equally necessitated by the realisation that I require my hormone replacement therapy (HRT) prescription refilled. The irony doesn't escape me. That I'm off to query breast lumps at the same time I want to get more HRT. With mainstream media full of conflicting opinions regarding HRT, I had always been a little hesitant about using it. Slightly wary of a product that messed with my hormones. But after years of terrible perimenopause symptoms, especially hot flushes and migraines, four years ago, reassured by my gynaecologist, I had commenced using it and subsequently, found it an enormous help, my headaches virtually disappearing. While my initial concerns haven't gone away, it hasn't stopped me renewing my prescription every six months.

It's mid-December 2021 and Australia is in the thick of another Covid scare when my appointment becomes due. Worldwide, Omicron has just come on the scene and Australia, a country that has managed to lockout Covid's worse, is completely terrified. It means that only necessary physical examination appointments are being made for face-to-face meetings with doctors and everyone in the surgery is socially distancing, well sanitised, and correctly masked when I'm ushered in to see a young Dr Taylor. Not all that long graduated, she oozes youth, health and confidence. She's also caring and efficient and while she raises her eyebrows at the HRT prescription asked for immediately after a referral to get my breast lumps checked, she complies. There's no examination, just the handing over of prescription and referral.

A week later and it's 22 December. Christmas is in three days' time and along with visiting the nearby larger town of Ballina to have a breast mammogram, then ultrasound; my priority is to finish my Christmas shopping. Tomorrow I'll head to the Gold Coast to collect my daughter Paige and Aunt Cherry, both of whom will spend Christmas with us. I'm in the Christmas spirit and much more concerned about the Christmas menu than I am about my upcoming tests.

It's a boiling day, the temperature is hovering in the high thirties, and thus the air-conditioned offices of North Coast Radiology are appreciated when, masked up, I take off my top for my mammogram. For those not aware, a mammogram is an x-ray picture of your breast. It's not a pleasant procedure as your breasts are squeezed tightly and individually between two cold metal plates and held there for an uncomfortable amount of time, while the x-ray is taken. For those with lumpy breasts, it's particularly painful. Often, I get a compassionate, gentle female; today the radiographer is Bill, an elderly solemn gentleman, but it doesn't take long before I am back in the waiting room awaiting my ultrasound. I've been waiting for probably five minutes when a nurse appears, asking if I could return to the mammogram room. Apparently, Bill wants to take a few more images of my left breast. I'm not concerned. It's not the first time I have had to have extra mammograms, plus, I pointed out the slightly dimpled area to him earlier. He's obviously just being extra vigilant.

Following this second mammogram, it's not much later that I am ushered in for my ultrasound. Unlike a mammogram, an ultrasound is generally non-invasive and painless. Using high-frequency sound waves, an internal body image is captured by a skilled sonographer running a gelled transductor, a small handheld device that resembles a microphone, over each breast. Today my sonographer seems very vigilant as he thoroughly runs the probe over first my right then, my left breast. By the time he has finished, I'm racing to get out of there and hit the shops.

A few hours later, and I get my first uncomfortable nudge that maybe this time everything is not exactly as it should be. I am driving home and my phone rings. It's Dr Taylor advising that North Coast Radiology have contacted her and are advising that I should have a breast biopsy at my earliest convenience. They have a vacancy at St Vincent's Hospital in Lismore tomorrow. Would I like it? Now I have been called back to have biopsies before, but never has the call back been so hurried and whilst a part of me knows that I probably should take this quick appointment, another part of me is saying 'Yeah, it's just another biopsy, it'll be the same result as before. And what about Christmas? What about collecting Paige from the Gold Coast train station tomorrow?' In this instance, Christmas wins, the whisper of fear is squashed and a later appointment for 7 January, two weeks later, is made. As she hangs up the phone, Dr Taylor does fire one parting piece of advice, 'Just to be cautious, can you stop taking the HRT?'

Christmas passes, memorable, by a welcoming last-minute relaxation of the severe Queensland and New South Wales border closure rules, extremely hot humid days and terrible headaches brought on by HRT withdrawal. Following a hysterectomy in 2020 and gall bladder removal in 2021, my body has taken a battering over the past few years and this Christmas with its hot days, doesn't help. I'm eating healthily, drinking little alcohol but still feeling worn.

Friday, 7 January and 8.45 am finds me at St Vincent's Hospital, Lismore. Because of Covid restrictions, my husband Darryl is not allowed to accompany me into the hospital so finds himself waiting in the car. The rain dripping against the windows and the rhythmic ticking of the blue solar powered dashboard elephant, his only distraction. St Vincent's Hospital has long been a stalwart institution of Lismore and its age is showing. Empty of visitors because of Covid, its peeling wallpaper, flaking paint and threadbare carpet are even more noticeable. It's awful enough that I make a deal with myself that if this breast thing does need to go further then, anything that needs doing from now on will be done at the much nicer John Flynn Hospital at Coolangatta. The same hospital where Darryl, 11 years ago following a horrific motor bike accident, spent three months recovering.

A second reason I don't want to be here at St Vincent's is because this is where Darryl's late mother, Barbara, spent the final few days of her life in the hospice ward. St Vincent's, to me, will always be synonymous with a grand lady dying.

'So, what's Bill seen then?' is the unexpected and slightly disconcerting greeting uttered by the sonographer as I make my way into a freezing room.

'Let's have a look.' Which he does once I have peeled off my top and uncomfortably reclined myself on a hard narrow paper lined bed.

'Mm,' muttered as he presses the transductor somewhat painfully over my left breast.

'I think I'll get Paul in to have a look. He's the radiographer and will be the one taking the actual biopsy.'

Like the sonographer, Paul is lovely and very attentive. As I lie on the table thinking how nice they both appear to be, Paul runs through the procedure.

'I'm going to first numb your breast, then, guided by ultrasound, will take two, maybe three samples of tissue using this hollow needle.

The procedure is called a core needle biopsy, and I'll end up with some plugs of tissue that will be used to identify whether there is anything nasty.'

The injection that numbs the biopsied site is more painful than the biopsy itself and after taking three 'plugs', I am free to go. As I make my way towards the door, the sonographer, lovely to the end, does advise me to make a follow-up appointment with my GP.

'Give them a call on Monday.'

Addendum

Symptoms – Of breast cancer can include:

A dimpling or pitting of the breast skin. A lump or thickening. Redness, inflammation or soreness. Abnormal discharge from the nipple. A change in the nipple appearance or a change in the size, shape or appearance of the breast itself.

CHAPTER
2

Cancer Types and Sub-Types

IN WHAT MUST BE A rarity these days, I have been going to the same doctor's office for the past 50 years. All but one of the doctors have changed, and it moved location once in those 50 years, but it's the same clinic. And for as long as I can remember, it's always had the same policy regarding follow-up appointments—don't phone us; if there is anything of importance, we will phone you. And so, two days later, on the following Monday, this is what I do, or rather, don't do.

'If there is something wrong, they will phone me,' I reassure both myself and Darryl. 'I've had biopsies before, and they never phoned, and everything was fine.'

While I'm slightly on edge and keeping to myself that the demeanour of both the sonographer and radiographer at St Vincent's was a little unusual, the lack of any phone call on Monday and Tuesday soon dispels any niggles of apprehension. To further cement the feeling that all is well, on Wednesday, five days after my biopsy, I return to my doctor's clinic to have a nurse administer my Covid booster. It occurs at twelve noon and they make no mention of biopsy results or follow-up appointments. As I make the 10-minute drive home to Brunswick Heads, arm aching slightly, I can't help feeling relieved. That tiny morsel of anxiety that's been swimming around has gone.

Unfortunately, that feeling of relief lasts a mere 20 minutes. The time it takes for me to make a sandwich, boil the jug, and take my first sip of my afternoon coffee.

'Hi Emma. I'm phoning to see if you have any results.'

It's Dr Taylor phoning me. To say I'm surprised is an understatement.

'No. I was waiting for a call from you,' I reply.

'Hold on then. I'll have a look now.'

As she takes a moment or two to look up my results, my thoughts are in rather a confused turmoil. I'm thinking—this is weird, Dr Taylor hasn't seen my results yet? How come? She asked if I had heard anything! Who from? This is not the way things normally happen. By the time she comes back onto the phone, I've decided that this is a strange way of going about things. I'm not sure I like it.

'Ok. Yes, I have them here… it's not very good news, I'm afraid. Could you come into the surgery this afternoon? Maybe bring someone with you.'

And that's all it takes for a life to change completely.

Funny enough, it's not the first time our life has completely changed. In 2011, Darryl, while travelling with a group of friends in Far North Queensland, was involved in a serious motor-bike accident. The result, after spending five months recovering in hospitals, was it left Darryl with various lifelong injuries, pain and an inability to work. If you're interested in knowing more, it's well documented in my book—*Bucket Lists and Walking Sticks*. Five years after his accident, to make life easier, we had downsized to a lovely townhouse in the seaside town of Brunswick Heads where, once the kids had left home and we weren't travelling, we would fill our days with activities such as lawn bowls. Darryl is at lawn bowls when I take that phone call that once again changes the trajectory of our life and hurries home to accompany me back to the doctor's surgery.

'Yes. It's breast cancer, I'm afraid, invasive lobular breast cancer,' says Dr Taylor an hour later.

I'm going to stop my story here for a bit to give a simplified overview of the types of breast cancer there are and their subtypes. Clarification of what that sentence—'It's invasive lobular breast cancer,' actually means. It's knowledge I didn't have before commencing my own journey and seeing as more and more of us are being diagnosed with or know someone who has been diagnosed with breast cancer, it's handy information to have. It will provide more context, more understanding, when next you hear that someone has breast cancer.

Breast Cancers are generally divided into two categories or types: non-invasive and invasive.

Non-Invasive Breast Cancer:

These are cancers that are contained within the breast lobules or milk ducts and have not invaded or grown into the surrounding breast tissue. They are called *carcinoma in situ,* the most common being.

- Ductal carcinoma in situ (DCIS) followed by:
- Lobular carcinoma in situ (LCIS).

Both types of cancer are non-life threatening, but they risk turning into invasive breast cancer later in life. Treatment options include lumpectomy (removal of the tumour and some normal surrounding tissue) or mastectomy (removal of the entire breast), usually followed by radiation therapy (targeted x-rays that can kill cancer).

Invasive Breast Cancer:

- Invasive breast cancers have spread outside the breast lobules or milk ducts and into the surrounding breast tissue. The three most common types of invasive breast cancer are:
- Invasive ductal carcinoma—accounting for roughly 70 to 80% of all cases, this is cancer that began in the milk ducts.
- Invasive lobular carcinoma—accounting for roughly 5 to 10% of cases, this is cancer that began in the milk-producing lobe of the breast.
- Inflammatory breast cancer—accounting for roughly 1 to 5% of cases, this cancer can occur in either the ducts or lobes and tends to spread faster than the other types.

Treatment options for invasive breast cancer are surgery (mastectomy, lumpectomy, lymph node removal), chemotherapy (the use of powerful drugs to kill cancer cells), radiation and therapies such as endocrine, biological and bisphosphonates (the use of drugs to block various causes of cancer growth).

Outside of non-invasive and invasive breast cancer, there are rarer types such as Paget's disease of the nipple, angiosarcoma of the breast and phyllodes tumours, but most diagnoses fall into either non-invasive or invasive.

Breast Cancer Subtypes:

Breast cancer subtypes describe the smaller groups that we can divide a type of cancer into based on certain cancer cell characteristics. Knowing the subtype of a cancer plays an important role in planning treatment and determining prognosis.

- The three main breast cancer subtypes are:
- Hormone receptor-positive breast cancer
- HER2 positive breast cancer
- Triple negative breast cancer

Hormone receptor-positive breast cancer

These are cancers that need the female hormones oestrogen and/or progesterone to grow and reproduce. About two-thirds of breast cancers are hormone receptor positive. Based on five-year relative survival percentages, hormone receptor positive cancers have a better prognosis than HER2 and triple negative.

HER2 positive breast cancer

These types of breast cancer have too much of a protein called Human Epidermal growth factor Receptor 2 on their surface compared to normal cells. This excess of HER2 receptors bolsters the growth of the cancer cells. HER2 positive cancer may be hormone receptor positive or negative and form around 20% of breast cancers.

Triple negative breast cancer

Triple negative breast cancer is probably the scariest to get diagnosed with. Triple negative breast cancer does not have any of the three common receptors found on breast cancer cells (oestrogen, progesterone or HER2) which makes it harder to treat. Approximately 15% of breast cancers are triple negative.

'And it appears to be hormone receptor positive,' Dr Taylor continues. 'But I've made an appointment for you for tomorrow afternoon with Dr Leong at John Flynn Hospital. She's a breast and endocrine specialist and, from what I've heard, a very good one. She'll be able to provide you with more information.'

While I'm not altogether surprised by Dr Taylor's words, the demeanour of the radiographer and sonographer at St Vincent's Hospital had provided some subconscious forewarning, and her earlier phone call had put me on high alert. I am surprised by how quickly everything is moving. A specialist's appointment tomorrow, less than 24 hours away, that's unheard of. Specialists normally take between three and six months to see. It's only sometime later do I learn why. That Australian law advises you be referred to a specialist within two weeks of a positive breast cancer diagnosis.

Addendum

Take someone with you to each of your appointments.

You're going to be inundated with information, unfamiliar terms, advice. You are more than likely not going to remember everything. Take someone with you who will not only be your memory but someone with whom you can later consult with. At the very least, take a notepad and pen or use notes on your phone.

CHAPTER

3

Meeting my Breast Surgeon

―――――――⟨∞⟩―――――――

THE FOLLOWING DAY, THE DAY of my breast specialist appointment, also happens to be my mother's birthday. Along with my sisters Michelle and Lucy, Darryl and I have organised to meet and celebrate mum's birthday in the garden of her retirement complex. It's a very low-key affair because of the ongoing Covid restrictions and while I have earlier made Michelle aware of my diagnosis, mum and Lucy are ignorant. They'll be informed once I have seen the specialist and have further news.

Dr Leong, when Darryl and I, accompanied by Michelle, who will be taking take notes, enter her offices some hours later, eventuates to be a wonderful pocket rocket of knowledge who projects confidence like a rock star. She's had a look through my clinical report and confirms that what I have is invasive lobular breast cancer, estrogen and progesterone positive.

'Lobular means that it started in the lobes of your breast, unlike the more common ductal carcinomas,' she reiterates. 'Only about 10-15% of all breast cancers are lobular. They can also be harder to detect. But hormone positive is good, we have more treatment options. Have you ever taken HRT?'

As I confess that yes, I have taken HRT periodically for headaches over the past couple of years, in the back of my mind I'm guiltily questioning (again), whether I should have. I know that no doctor is ever going to denounce HRT, but along with Dr Taylors' earlier insistence that I cease taking it immediately, I'm beginning to strongly wonder if there is a link between HRT and my current diagnosis. A suspicion that unfortunately, I'll probably never get an answer for.

Following a few more probing questions and a brief physical breast examination, Dr Leong then outlines what needs to happen next.

'First step will be a breast MRI, which will help determine how much cancer there is. It's invasive, which means it has spread from your breast lobule, so you will need chemotherapy. I would also advise a mastectomy. You could have chemotherapy first or a mastectomy. It's up to you.'

'I want a mastectomy first. I want it out of my body. Actually, I want both breasts taken.' I reply.

'I don't advocate having both breasts removed unless necessary,' Dr Leong answers. 'You'll probably need five months of chemotherapy and maybe radiation treatment afterwards. That will be up to your oncologist. It will make it easier going through treatment having just the one wound to contend with.'

'Would you recommend a PET scan?' Michelle interjects. Being an occupational therapist and married to an anaesthetist, she will always campaign for the most comprehensive treatment. 'I mean, if it was your sister sitting here, would you suggest a more thorough test than just an MRI?' she pushes.

After some thought, Dr Leong replies. 'Yes, if it was my sister here, then I would opt for a PET scan as well.'

'Ok.' I summarise. 'MRI and PET scans, then mastectomy. When would chemotherapy start?'

'Chemotherapy usually begins within four weeks of your mastectomy. Again, it will be up to your oncologist.'

'What about reconstruction?' Michelle asks.

'At this stage, I'm not interested,' I reply. 'I don't want to go through further operations.'

'You have time to give it more thought,' says Dr Leong.

'Think about nice perky breasts,' says Michelle.

'I'll think about it, but at this stage, I'm not interested.'

Leaving Dr Leong's office, and testament once again to how quickly things can progress following a breast cancer diagnosis, my phone rings before I've even reached the car. It's South Coast Radiology wishing to book my MRI appointment for the following Monday afternoon. In four days' time. And if it's convenient, my PET scan will be early Tuesday morning.

Armed with a little more information and slightly more aware of what lies ahead, the next step is probably going to be a tough one. Informing my family and friends. At this stage, only Darryl and Michelle are aware of my diagnosis. As I sit that night with Darryl, trying to determine who to tell first and how much to tell them, I realise with dismay that it's even more difficult than I was expecting. Harder than actually learning I have breast cancer. How do you tell your mother or children, without causing them too much alarm, that you have something that may kill you and you are now in for the fight of your life. And what order will cause the least offence—mother first, followed by children or children first? As our son Pierce walks into the room as we are sitting discussing this choice, the decision is made for us.

Pierce is an old soul, a deep thinker, who has been living with us for the past four years whilst he undertook an electrical apprenticeship. Recently graduated, he'll only be with us a few more weeks before moving to the Gold Coast where he'll look for work as a qualified tradesperson. True to his nature, he takes the news quietly. The questions, and there will be a lot of them, will come once he has fully absorbed the information. I phone Paige, our daughter, next. About to begin her third year studying for a social work degree and with a nursing certificate already under her belt, her questions are broad and probing. It's quite reassuring to talk with her, and I know she will always be a comfort.

The hardest conversation of all comes the following morning, and that is with my mother. She is shopping at Aldi when I phone her, and although I should wait until a more appropriate time, I chicken out and just blurt the news to her. I don't really give her any choice but to hold herself together while she continues with her shopping. Later, she tells me she had to keep stopping herself from crying as she pushed her trolley up and down the aisles.

After that, it becomes easier. Darryl and I visit my stepmother Patma, and Darryl's father Lloyd, both of whom have lost partners to cancer, understand the cancer highway and thus take the news stoically. Friends are informed, as are my lawn bowls compatriots. Some are wonderful and incredibly reassuring with their response, knowing exactly how to reply, others, as I tell Darryl.

'Have no idea how to react.'

A surprising thing I do learn is that nearly everyone I talk to knows someone who has or has had, breast cancer.

Advising people of my diagnosis keeps me busy, anaesthetises me temporarily to the reality of my situation but over the following days, this changes and it begins to sink in that things will never be the same again. Outwardly, I still look the same, but internally, my thoughts begin to fester and all I can think about—10, 20, 30 times a day—is I have cancer. I'm going to lose a breast. I'm going to have chemotherapy. Suddenly my health and body have taken on a whole new level of concern. So much so that when my lymph nodes swell and my arm continues to ache from my Covid booster, I am so paranoid it's making the cancer worse that I phone Dr Leong's office. She phones back, reassuring me that all is fine. Covid also becomes much more concerning. Not only because of what it could do to me if I caught it, but how it could prevent upcoming treatments, appointments, and operations if I become even a close contact. We already had some hand sanitiser and masks in the house. Now we get a whole lot more and make up a well-stocked hygiene station near our front door. Pierce, going out to work each day, could potentially bring Covid back with him. To mitigate any exposure, we make a temporary kitchen in the garage and Pierce finds himself confined to his bedroom, bathroom and the garage for the remainder of his time with us.

Ten years ago, about a year after Darryl's accident, we found ourselves attending countless doctors' and solicitors' appointments. To make these meetings more enjoyable, especially those some distance away, we created a practice that we called 'medical tourism'—an excuse to spend the night away from home, somewhere close to the appointment. With my breast MRI scheduled for the Monday afternoon at Robina, a 50-minute drive from Brunswick Heads, and my PET scan pencilled in for early the following Tuesday at John Flynn Hospital, it's the perfect opportunity to have a medical holiday.

'We haven't been anywhere since we returned from our trip around the world,' I remind Darryl. 'We haven't been able to because of Covid. We could stay the night at Coolangatta, close to John Flynn. That way, you won't have to wait in the car near the hospital. Just drop me off, then return to the hotel. We'll be careful, wear masks and use sanitiser. It would be nice to get something good out of all of this. Do something fun.' The trip I am referring to is a four-month adventure that had us circumnavigating the entire globe. It's documented in my book *Itchy Feet & Bucket Lists*. Despite the circumstances, I'm eager for any excuse to once again get away.

'You should be finished before I'm due to check-out of the hotel,' Darryl replies. 'I'm not all that keen to stay somewhere at the moment with Covid, but I know you'll enjoy it.'

Addendum

Be prepared - When meeting with any new medical practitioners, you may be asked to complete paperwork. Have answers to common questions—i.e. what medications or supplements you are taking, Medicare and health fund details—handy.

CHAPTER

4

MRIs, CTs and PET Scans

AN MRI IS A NON-INVASIVE procedure that uses magnetic fields and radio waves to take a cross examination of your body. Amongst other things, it can detect breast tumours, measure their size and show if they have spread.

I've had an MRI before, in this same building actually. It was to ascertain the size and location of my uterus prior to a hysterectomy. That was early 2020, pre-Covid exhaustion, and everyone was jovial, and we could see their faces. Today, as I sit waiting for my name to be called, everyone is fully masked, there are fewer patients, and no one seems friendly. Like last time, the room with the MRI scanner is freezing, as stripped down to my undies and with a paper gown draped around me, I am directed towards the large donut-shaped machine with a retractable table protruding from it. Unlike last time where I lay on my back having my tummy scanned, this time I lay on my stomach with my breasts hanging. It's much scarier lying this way. I feel trapped, more vulnerable, and I am thankful that I am not claustrophobic. I have earphones on, and the piped music masks the awful banging, thumping, and clicking noise the machine makes as my body is fed through the donut. Halfway through the procedure, a dye is injected into the cannula (a thin tube inserted into my vein to administer any medication) that has been inserted into my right arm and I get a metallic taste in the back of my throat while warmth floods my groin, both sensations I have been warned to expect. Thankfully, the whole procedure lasts less than 30 minutes and we are free to make our way to Coolangatta where, despite Covid's pall, we enjoy our medical tourism night at the Mantra hotel.

I'm not allowed to eat before the following morning's PET scan, so it's fortunate that it's an early appointment. I've never had a PET scan before, so I'm grateful that a technician takes the time to step me through it.

'You're here for a PET scan with contrast, which means first of all, I will inject a small amount of radioactive substance into your arm. We'll then leave you resting in this comfortable recliner for about an hour or so while the liquid works its way around your bloodstream before taking you in for your PET scan.'

'And the PET scan will detect the radioactive liquid?' I question.

'That's right. The solution is just a simple sugar that's been joined with a radioactive substance which should accumulate in the body where more energy is given off. Cancer cells are fast dividing, thus they give off more energy. The sugar syrup should accumulate in these areas and be detectable by the PET scanner.'

'And how long will the PET scan take?'

'The scan itself should take no more than 30 minutes.'

After once again stripping to my undies and cloaking myself in a paper gown, an intravenous line is inserted into a vein on the back of my hand, a liquid is injected, and I am left in front of a television for the next hour and a half. Sitting here, flipping through the channels, warmed by a cosy blanket and far removed from the Covid world and worries outside, I'm thinking, this isn't too bad. The scan which follows is low key as well. It involves another narrow, flat table that feeds into a noodle like tunnel and this time I'm on my back with my arms raised above my head. As promised, it takes only 30 minutes and two days later Darryl, Michelle and I are back to Dr Leong's office to get the results of both tests.

'While scans can be useful,' Dr Leong mutters while scrolling through her screen, analysing my results, 'sometimes they can just complicate matters. In your case, it appears to be the latter. The MRI is inconclusive. While there is a poorly defined breast mass at 12 o'clock, I cannot ascertain its size or clinical staging. And the PET scan. Although there are no hot spots anywhere, there is a meningioma in your left sinus and a slight thickening of your chest cavity on your sternum. We'll monitor both. A brain MRI in about a month and a chest CT later. In about three months.'

'You said there are no hot spots anywhere,' I query her. 'How about the tumour in the left breast?'

'No, that's not showing up on the PET scan.'

'Not at all?' Darryl interjects.

'No. Unfortunately, PET scans don't always show everything. We'll know more after the mastectomy, which I would like to schedule for next week—28 January. You'll also be having a sentinel node biopsy and maybe an axillary lymph node dissection.'

As I'm trying to fathom how the PET scan has failed to detect a cancer we know is there, and dismally realise that it may have missed others, Dr Leong is continuing. 'Prior to your operation, you will have a blue dye injected into your left breast, which will help me locate the sentinel node, the first node that the cancer may have spread to. Once I have removed this node, or in some cases, nodes, a pathologist will inspect it under a microscope, while you're still on the operating table. If it comes back positive, I'll have to do an axillary node dissection which involves removing all the nodes in the armpit just in case they also contain cancer. You'll know as soon as you wake up whether I have had to do the dissection. If you wake up with one drain, I've only had to do the sentinel node biopsy. If you wake up with two drains, then the sentinel node was positive for cancer, and I have also had to do an axillary lymph node dissection.'

Sitting sometime later in the hospital coffee shop, the atmosphere is a little lighter. Flabbergasting and concerning as it is that the PET scan hasn't even revealed my known tumour, at least I have a date for its removal.

'It's the same date that our house in Mullumbimby settles', I remind Darryl. 'Let's hope it all goes smoothly as we won't be much help.'

To complicate things slightly, a month prior to my diagnosis, we had accepted an offer on an investment property we held in the nearby town of Mullumbimby. Like many countries around the world, Covid has caused property prices to rise in Australia and after months of indecision, we had finally decided to take advantage of the increase and sell the property.

'Maybe the timing is perfect,' Darryl replies. 'We can just leave it all up to the agents, not worry about any of it and when you wake up from your operation, it should all be settled and over.'

The following eight days before my mastectomy are quite conflicting. Increasingly worried about catching Covid, Darryl and I find ourselves rarely leaving the house and Pierce, with his comings and goings, is made to feel even more like a potential disease carrying interloper. Lawn bowls, previously a major source of our entertainment are out of the question for the foreseeable future, as is shopping or visiting friends. Surprisingly, I spend more time than expected thinking over whether I should have a reconstruction or not. One of my old school friends, Michelle, had a double mastectomy a few years back, and her opinion regarding reconstruction and other things proves invaluable, reminding me that some choices don't need to be rushed.

'Personally, I decided against reconstruction,' she had advised. 'I didn't want to put myself through any more operations. Just take your time with any important decisions and, most importantly, look after yourself. Put yourself first.'

On one of the eight days, an amazing hamper arrives from Paige. Full of toiletries, protein bars, slippers, glasshouse candle, pillow, chocolate, bath bombs, hand sanitizer, thermometer, masks, and goodness know what else, it's the best hamper I have ever seen, let alone received and I have the most fun since my diagnosis, unpacking and using the items.

Disordinate as they are, the days are not nearly so bad as the nights. Since the onset of perimenopause five years ago, I've found a full night's sleep difficult, often waking and lying for hours, my mind plotting, planning, unable to get back to sleep. Whereas not so long ago, these main night-time thoughts were simple—whether I could handle the freezing temperature of a Mongolian Ger, where to travel to next or how to improve my bowling—my current thinking is a lot different, a lot more complex. Lying wide awake, nightmare thoughts regarding my diagnosis flood my mind and I can't stop it from its depressing questioning. Will I be here in one, five, ten years' time? What will happen to Darryl and the kids if I die? Should I have reconstruction? How bad will chemotherapy be? Am I going to lose my hair?

Finally, thankfully, the agonising wait is over. It's time to start the fight. Stepping out of the shower on the eve of my operation, I eyeball my left breast with its innocuous looking dimple, marvelling how something so innocent looking can be so terrible. I also gloomily wonder what I am going to look like once the breast has gone.

Addendum

Ask for copies (electronic and/or hardcopies) of all your reports and test results—for example x-rays, scans, blood work. Keep electronic copies in a folder on your phone. More than once, I have been able to instantly provide a specialist with a relevant document saving time and providing immediate answers. Some radiology organisations allow you to access your scans and reports via an app on your phone. Enquire.

CHAPTER

5

Sentinel Node Biopsy

THE SUN HAS BARELY RISEN when Darryl bracingly wishes me goodbye and good luck at the drop-off point to John Flynn Hospital. Because of Covid's restrictions, I won't see him again for a few days and he's not happy about it. Personally, I'm looking forward to some alone time, to gathering my thoughts and focusing on no one else but myself. Before I check into the hospital, I present myself at nearby South Coast Radiology. I'm here for sentinel node mapping. During my actual mastectomy, my sentinel node, the first lymph node that the cancer may have spread to, will be removed for analysis. Using a special substance containing a small amount of radioactivity that flows towards the lymph nodes, the mapping this morning will pinpoint its exact location. It will be the node with the highest amount of radioactivity. The procedure doesn't take very long and, armpit now full of strange marks, I leave the radiology department and check in to John Flynn Hospital.

Like when I was admitted previously for my hysterectomy and gallbladder operations, the first order of procedure is a Covid test. Fortunately, it's negative and permits me access to my pre-operative assessment where I'm measured, weighed, forced into compression stockings, another paper gown and then left with all the other patients waiting to have an operation. As I wait, I can't help but be impressed, moved even, with the passing nursing staff. I'm not sure if it's because of these strange Covid times, but every staff member who walks past me either offers a hot blanket or a word of encouragement. Some give me a little pat on the shoulder and one squeezes both of my hands while reassuring me that all will be good. Whatever the reason, it's very pacifying and by the time I'm eventually wheeled down to the operation theatre, I am ready.

The bits from theatre that I remember before passing out are interesting. For the first time ever, I walk into the operating room and clamber onto the table under my own steam. It's a huge glaringly lit area, freezing cold, with many people buzzing around. As I lie on what could pass for a padded plank, compression cuffs painfully squeezing my legs, my left breast marked with a distinctive arrow, Dr Leong speaks to me.

'Just to explain once again that we will do a sentinel node biopsy and a left breast mastectomy. If the node comes back positive, I'll do an axillary lymph node dissection. You'll know as soon as you wake up whether I have had to do the dissection. If you wake up with one drain, I've only had to do the sentinel node biopsy. If you wake up with two drains, then the sentinel node or nodes were positive for cancer, and I had to carry out an axillary node dissection as well.'

As the anaesthetist checks with me that I'm feeling ok, and I'm thinking just hurry up and put me under, everything goes black.

'How many drains are there?' A clock high on the wall shows that it's 5 pm. I've been asleep for hours, and a nurse is hovering over me.

'Just the one.'

'Are you sure? Really sure? Only one?'

'Yes. Just one. How are you feeling? How's the pain? Do you need something?'

'Definitely one?'

As I finally start to believe what the nurse is telling me, I have only the one drain, I try to concentrate on exactly what she is asking me. How am I feeling? Incredibly relieved actually, now that the overwhelming worry of knowing whether the cancer has spread to the sentinel node has been answered. And sore. Really sore, to be honest.

'I don't feel as bad as I did after my hysterectomy,' I eventually answer the nurse. 'But I am sore.'

As she tops up my drip with painkiller and finds an ice block for me to suck, I'm feeling sad about my missing breast, uncomfortable and in pain, but more than anything, unbelievably relieved. One drain—yes! The cancer hasn't spread beyond my breast.

Perhaps one of the best things about John Flynn Hospital is its location. Situated on a small hill close to Coolangatta airport, many of its rooms and offices offer incredible views of planes gently gliding into land, with the mesmerising Pacific Ocean as a backdrop. Wheeled a short time later by a wardsman into a room with a jaw dropping vista even better than I was expecting, I'm glad it's mine alone for the next two days. If I must be here, in pain, minus a breast, then I'm glad I have a stunning scene to look at.

And it's a scene that does help as, over the next two days, I start to recover and learn to accommodate life with a mono-boob chest. I was advised beforehand to bring button up pyjamas and I am grateful

I listened. With my torso tightly bound in what feels like a broad rubber band; a suction pump and a tube draining bloody fluid, hanging uncomfortably from my left armpit, it's nearly impossible to lift my arms, so button up tops are mandatory. I'm a bit surprised by my bindings. Dr Leong had warned me about the drain and the suction pump, but I hadn't given her words much thought. Now, I can't believe how uncomfortable everything is. Showering is particularly tricky, requiring body contortions to get wet without unduly affecting the hanging paraphernalia.

Luckily, along with the view, the nursing staff are fantastic. One of these is Lesley, a breast care nurse. Not a McGrath breast care nurse, I've been advised that the entire Gold Coast area doesn't have any of these, unfortunately, but a dedicated breast care nurse, nonetheless. She's specially trained to manage the care of those with breast cancer and she's a godsend. Teaching me how to empty my drain, providing generously donated cushions and a bag that I can use to hide the gory appendage hanging from me, and most helpful of all, linking me to websites with others going through this same thing.

At some stage, a physiotherapist visits with a list of exercises I'm to do for the next six months. As she steps me through them, I'm shocked at how limited the mobility is in my upper left arm. I recovered quite quickly from my hysterectomy and gallbladder operations through daily yoga and exercise. I know the only way I'm going to get through this mastectomy is through following this physio routine.

I'm in Ward 3B—Women's health. I know there are others out there going through what I am, I see them when I go for my frequent walks around the ward. Their drainage tubes identify them, but, along with our visitors, it's something Covid has taken from us. We are unable to mix and share our stories. The best we can do is have Lesley and the other nurses pass on any useful information.

It's a quiet Sunday afternoon when I am discharged. Dr Leong rockets in beforehand to check that I am fine to leave and reminds me I have an appointment in her offices this coming Thursday. 'My nurse will take the pump off. The drain will probably need to stay a little longer, and we'll have the final pathology report back from your operation. I removed three lymph nodes, all of which looked clear. So, while it appears as if your cancer has been contained to your breast only, the report will confirm it.'

While I'm happy to be leaving hospital, I'm also slightly stressed. Hospital offers safety and security with your every need met. Now I'm on my own. Although one thing that does manage to cheer me up is that our bank account is looking very rosy. It appears that despite us being totally absent, settlement on our Mullumbimby house went smoothly.

January 2022 has been a wet summer and the following days, as it absolutely teams with rain, I find myself watching plenty of television or reading up on breast cancer in between performing my physio exercises. My reading has revealed that it looks as if I may have been even luckier than I had thought. Unlike ductal breast cancers, which I learn, form in detectable lumps, lobular cancer grows in lines.

'Or like a spider web,' I say to Darryl. 'Because it grows like a web, it's really difficult to detect, especially if you have dense breast tissue like me. Mammograms hardly ever detect it—it may even have been missed during my 2020 appointment. It is usually detected through ultrasound or MRI, and by the time it is discovered, it is often quite advanced. I think I have been very lucky.'

'Did you say lobular doesn't show up in mammograms?'

'It rarely shows up in mammograms,' I correct. 'Scary, hey. Here we are, told to have regular scans which may not even detect a cancer which is there.'

Pierce has now moved out of home, so the worry of him bringing Covid into the house has fortunately gone. We have also taken to ordering all our groceries online. Despite the discomfort of my tight bandages and drain, I'm sleeping well, a combination of the huge U-shape pillow that came with Paige's hamper and the Endone prescribed by Dr Leong. By Wednesday, five days post-surgery, I've even learnt how to shower proficiently despite the tube and bag that hangs from my body. This doesn't mean, Thursday morning, that I'm not itching to have my pump removed, the bandage loosened and maybe, the drain taken out.

Addendum

Hospital Kit - The average stay in hospital following a mastectomy is 1-3 nights. Ensure you have at least two sets of pyjamas with button up tops as fluid leakage can occur. Pyjamas that double as day attire are good. Dressing gown. Toiletries. Medications. Slippers. Phone. Long phone charger. Additional bag to bring things home in.

CHAPTER

6

Mastectomy

———————— ⟨⟩ ————————

IT'S STILL POURING WITH RAIN as we make the 50-minute drive back to John Flynn Hospital. I'm a nervous passenger, so Darryl takes it slowly. Amongst the many conversations we have as we travel, is what to do with the funds from our Mullumbimby property.

'Maybe invest in a rental property up here,' I laughingly suggest. 'It would make hospital visits easier.'

We are early, so pop into the coffee shop for a bracing beverage before making our way to Dr Leong's office. Here, much to my relief, both the pump and bandage are removed, and I get my first look at my new torso with its single boob and adjacent horizontal scar. I would still have preferred a double mastectomy, a little more uniformity, but maybe this doesn't look so bad.

'The drain will need to stay longer,' says Skye, the nurse. 'And Dr Leong also has your full pathology results.'

'Hi,' Dr Leong utters as she powers into the room, report in her hand.

'It's not as good as I was hoping, I'm afraid. I'm really surprised. Follow up pathology found five tumours in your left breast. 0.5 mm, 1 mm, 2 mm, 14 mm and 52 mm.'

'You mean 5.2 mm,' Darryl interrupts.

'No. 52 mm', Dr Leong reiterates.

'Over 5 cm' Darryl says incredulously.

'Yes. And invasive lobular carcinoma was found in all three of the lymph nodes we removed.' She shakes her head. 'All three! And none of them showed positive in the original testing. Unfortunately, it means I'm going to have to operate again. I'll have to go in and do an axillary lymph node clearance or dissection. If you wish, I can also offer a right breast mastectomy at the same time.'

The news is so overwhelming that I'm just sitting there speechless, trying to absorb it all. The size and number of tumours have gone over my head, I'll leave it to Darryl to clarify those for me later, but I do grasp that my cancer has spread outside of my breast, into my lymph nodes and my thoughts of just moments ago are being answered. I am being offered a right breast mastectomy. Something that I wanted from the beginning.

'Yes, I want a right breast mastectomy. It will take away the fear that the cancer may be in this breast also, or it may occur in this breast at a later stage.'

'Ok. I'll get my receptionist to book you in for next week. Wednesday.'

'Great. Do you also do an axillary lymph node dissection on the right side?'

'No. With an axillary node clearance, there is a large risk of lymphoedema. We wouldn't want to take the nodes from both sides unless absolutely necessary.'

My mother lives a 10-minute drive from the hospital, and we are due to visit her next. We are both feeling quite stunned and use the drive time to pull ourselves together. One of the main thoughts running through my head is that I now know what I want to do with our investment money. I definitely want to move up here closer to my mother and sister and the hospital.

We make it a quick visit. Mum's currently going through her own health issues. Recently diagnosed with chronic obstructive pulmonary disease (COPD), she's looking skinny, has developed a debilitating itch and has trouble breathing. Despite her own health concerns, she has an enormous bag of food for me. We leave without going into too much detail regarding my pathology results. They are too stressful.

That afternoon, we struggle again with who and in what order, do we tell this latest news. We had all thought that, although serious, I had dodged the bigger cancer bullet. That's now changed. My cancer is obviously going to have a larger effect on our lives than we originally thought. Maybe have serious consequences, so family and friends need to be updated. Being a mother, it's incredibly difficult telling my children. I'm supposed to be the adult. The strong one. Pierce and Paige are both quiet when we eventually gather ourselves enough to phone. They both phone back a few hours later with more questions but overall are positive and understanding, the resilience of youth. I am currently the president of our local women's lawn bowls club—the Brunswick Heads Women's Bowling Club. Knowing that I'm going to need every bit of time, energy and strength to fight this cancer battle, that evening I reluctantly resign from my presidency.

I have six days before I need to return to the hospital. Paige, who is currently studying at university and living in Brisbane, comes to stay for a few days and we spend time reorganising the upstairs of our house and cleaning out Pierce's room. He's left it in an awful mess. I later discover that reorganising and tidying are common among those who have just undergone a cancer diagnosis. It's called nesting apparently, and it's me trying to regain some control over my life.

While last week I just wanted to recover indoors, to hide away, this week I spend a lot of time going for long healing walks. I've always used walking as a means of clearing my head and stretching my body, and Brunswick Heads, with its river and beaches, is the perfect place to do this. It's on one of these healing jaunts that I decide to write this book. While I have recently discovered many self-help breast cancer manuals, I've yet to find a book that simply tells what happens when someone gets diagnosed. My book, I decide, will be my story that I hope newly diagnosed breast cancer survivors and others can read to learn what lies ahead.

Along with my walks, I persevere with physiotherapy on my left arm and wonder what I'm going to look and feel like once I have two breasts removed. An old school friend, Fiona, has learnt of my diagnosis on the local grapevine and sends amazing words of encouragement. Cards arrive and my sister-in-law Davina sends a gorgeous bunch of flowers. I'm not used to being someone with a serious ailment and over time, as I try to go about my life, I learn something. That it's better to acknowledge someone when they are going through something like this. I always feel much better after talking with people who offer their condolences than I do with those who just see me, then skulk away.

We use one of these six days to return to Coolangatta to look at a dual key investment unit. More than ever now, I want to move closer to the security of a hospital and Darryl can understand my concern. The unit is privately listed, and my drain is discreetly tucked into a bag under my arm as, fully masked, we walk through both apartment and studio. While it looks great and would be ideal, offering an investment as well as a home for us, I know that dual key properties are popular. If it's meant to be, then it will be, I think to myself as we journey back to Brunswick Heads.

One afternoon, a text arrives from one of my lawn bowling friends asking me to step outside. A few minutes later, a minibus arrives and members of my bowls pennants team spill from it, yelling and cheering. They have just won the regional pennants competition so will be off to State. It's a monumental event for our tiny club and while I am so happy and excited for them all, I can't help feeling jealous. I should have been there with them; I should be going to State. I'm going to have to get used to cancer robbing me of things.

On 9 February, the day of my second mastectomy operation, I wake early and go for a long cathartic walk along the Brunswick Heads break wall. While my chest area still feels sore and uncomfortable, the rest of my body feels good. It seems unfair that just when I'm starting to really recover from my first operation, I'm now subjecting my body to a second.

With this being my fifth operation in less than two years, I am very familiar with the pre-operation procedure. Covid test, weigh-in, compression stockings, gown, wait. This time, as I sit in the waiting room, I still have my phone with me as I am negotiating the purchase of that dual key unit. We have just put an offer in and are waiting for it to be accepted or a counteroffer suggested. My head is all over the place with my upcoming surgery, but at least this wheeling and dealing is taking my mind off the scary things.

Again I walk into the operating theatre under my own steam and this time when I wake, that conveniently placed clock is registering 9 pm. I've been unconscious for nearly eight hours. Again, a wards person wheels me to my room, not quite as good a view as last time, but incredible all the same. All is silent. It's a Wednesday night, and lying in my narrow bed, compression pumps working furiously on my legs, I cannot help thinking of what others, friends and family, may be doing on this weekday night. Training, restaurant, pub, tv. Anywhere, but in a hospital, I hope.

Lesley, the breast care nurse, is on duty, and along with a gift bag of goodies, has a funky fresh bag for me. This is for the new drain and pump that adorns my right-hand side and mirrors the drain still hanging from my left. These handmade bags, along with beanies, blankets, and little satin cushions I can rest under my arm to protect my scarred chest, are made by volunteers and it's hard to convey just how gratefully received they are.

Having slept for most of the day, it's a long, drawn-out night. Every hour or so, nursing staff come and check my temperature, heart rate and oxygen levels. I'm usually a side sleeper and now, with drains, pump and stitches on both sides of my torso, can only lie on my back. I suspect this will be the case for quite some time. Finally, in the very early hours, I manage to drift off.

It's not for long. Early each morning sees a changeover of nursing staff in hospital and their chatter soon wakes me up. Not long later and Dr Leong comes bursting in, exclaiming as she does so.

'What an operation. There was so much scar tissue from last week's mastectomy. Taking off your right breast was easy. But removing all the nodes from amongst the scar tissue in your left arm was very difficult.

That's why it took so long. It went well and we'll have the pathology back in a few days.'

That first morning after my second mastectomy, and it doesn't take long to realise that life and recuperation are going to be a bit harder this time around. I've now got two surprisingly long wounds to contend with, and the deep and painful lymph node dissection of my left armpit has totally scuppered any gains made with exercise following my first operation. I'm also, once again, tightly wrapped in an awful plastic bandage. So tightly wrapped that it feels as if my circulation has stopped, and my arms are slowly being cut off. I'm very grateful for the four hourly dose of painkillers.

Understanding, that physio and exercise are one of the few things I have control over and knowing they can only help me recover quicker, I spend a lot of my time walking laps of the ward and following the arm exercise routine I was given last time. I'm always masked up and again I lament Covid preventing me from mixing with the other ladies and one gentleman, going through this same thing. Despite having to design a convoluted hanging system in the bathroom in order to keep my bags dry and my drains free, shower time becomes a welcome time of day. I'm finding that the hot water on my plastic wrapped torso eases some of the pressure and relieves the pain. The compression stockings, or TEDS as they are called, drive me crazy, but I'm not allowed to take them off. A fact I discover when a nurse crossly orders me to put them back on. Although after night two, I balk at the noisy machine that pins me to the bed as it compresses my calf muscles. It's a barbaric machine designed to prevent sleep and so I refuse to use it.

Like with my first mastectomy, I develop painful little blisters under my plastic wrap and keep the nurses busy attending to them. They must make tiny incisions into the plastic to reach the blisters, then patch them using what appears to be a magic blister band-aid. Whatever it is,

I wished I had known about it when I was younger and often got blisters from inappropriate shoes.

I become an expert at clearing my drains and emptying my pouches and one afternoon the cannula administering my post-op medications, falls out. Despite three attempts from a nurse, she can't find a vein to attach a new one, so a cannula specialist is called. Although he disconcerts me somewhat by breathing all over me whilst not wearing a mask, he manages to fit a new one on the first attempt.

What all this does is cement the feeling that I do not want to return to hospital. I don't want any more operations. Five in two years is enough. I've been giving reconstruction further thought and have done a little research. Dr Leong has also mentioned some of my options. From what I can understand, I have two choices. Implant reconstruction, where my breasts would be rebuilt using implants such as silicon or saline. Or flap (also known as DIEP) reconstruction, where they would be rebuilt using tissue from elsewhere on my body.

With the implant option, I'll require another operation to insert what is called a tissue expander under the skin on either side of my chest. Over a period, these tissue expanders will be systematically filled with saline solution to stretch the skin, probably done at my surgeon's office. Eventually, anywhere between two and eighteen months later, they will have dilated enough for the expanders to be removed, again under anaesthetic, and replaced with implants.

The second option requires an operation to recreate two new breasts using skin, fat and blood vessels from either my abdomen, back, thigh or buttocks. Whichever part of my body the tissue is taken from will be the texture and colour of my new breasts. What both choices will leave me with are two completely numb breasts devoid of nipple and areola. If I want nipples and areolas, I can either opt for yet two more operations, as these are usually done separately, or find a skilled tattoo artist. My thoughts fly back to my sister Michelle's comment in Dr Leong's office 'you can have perky new breasts.' Well, ok, they may be new and if I choose implants, then they may be perky, but either way, they'll also be numb with strange nipples, and while the second option is the most natural using my own body parts, they'll never look nor feel like normal breasts. It's when I fully understand this that I make my decision. I'll remain flat and will be happy and proud to do so. I'll never have to wear another bloody uncomfortable bra ever again.

With my mastectomies out of the way, the next stage of my breast cancer journey, or, as I am starting to call it, my breast cancer adventure, will be chemotherapy, which, fortunately, can also be done here at John Flynn Hospital. To help me begin to understand what chemotherapy will entail, I am visited by Korin, one of the hospital's cancer care co-ordinators. Korin is a calm, elegant lady who I will later come to appreciate immensely. Today, she just loads me up with pamphlets and booklets.

My final day in hospital and it's marked by two events. The first is noticing one of my neighbours, a lady also adorned with drainage bags, being prepped again for surgery. She opted for a reconstruction apparently, has now caught an infection and is being wheeled back to theatre to have something done. I'm not sure what. I feel immensely sorry for her and not for the first time, realise just how much a breast cancer patient can go through. The second event occurs as I am waiting for the lift that will deposit me at the exit door of the hospital. A bell starts ringing, signalling the arrival of a newborn baby in the adjacent maternity ward. For days, pain, infection and disease have surrounded me. It's incredibly uplifting to hear that bell, knowing that it signifies life, happiness and health. I can't help a huge smile plastering my face.

Addendum

Find a good support network - The best piece of advice I can offer is to find an existing support network who can guide you, assist you, support you. I found (via *Facebook*) the *Women's Cancer Support - GC* group, created and facilitated by an amazing warrior called Sandra. Additionally, find yourself a breast care nurse. They are the experts and invaluable as you start to tread the breast cancer path.

CHAPTER

7

Infection

———⁓———

AS HAS BEEN TRUE FOR most of January and February, it's raining when Darryl collects me. He's incredibly glad to see me, drainage bags and all, although he comments I look as if I have lost some weight.

'I don't have an appetite,' I reply. 'I think it's the painkillers. It happened with my hysterectomy. I weighed nearly 70 kilograms before that operation. Then, following that and my gall bladder operation, it went down to 65 kilos. Now my mastectomies. I think I'm about 61 kilos. I probably lost about 500 grams with each breast.' I grin. I'm happy to be going home.

As mentioned earlier, for the past few weeks, to make life easier, our groceries have been delivered and that evening while Darryl uses these to cook dinner, I go through the bag of goodies given to me by Lesley the breast care nurse and the paperwork provided by Korin. Lesley's package is more fun. It contains sample sized lipsticks and perfumes, along with some scarves, all generously donated and there to make someone who has just lost a vital part of themselves feel a little better. There's also another little satin pillow that I can wear over my shoulder which will protect my chest wound, some fillable mastectomy bras (special bras with hollow pockets that can be stuffed) and even an example of this stuffing—a pair of hand knitted knockers (breasts). Korin's paperwork is extensive and informative. Along with information on lymphoedema (which sounds terrifying) and how to identify it, I find pamphlets on wigs and information on where to turn to for cancer support. The online cancer support groups interest me the most and I spend an hour or so joining Korin's suggested organisations alongside others I discover myself. While the *Women's Cancer Support - GC* group will end up being the most useful to me, others, *Breast Cancer Support Australia—for women, Breast Cancer Integrative Healing, Jane McLelland Off Label Drugs for Cancer, Healing Cancer Study Support Group, Verzenio Support Group, Lobular Breast Cancer, ILC Sisters, Fierce, FLAT, Forward,* will all later, play their part in my breast cancer adventure.

The following few days and it appears as if the rain will never stop. It's probably fortunate timing, as along with a bout of diarrhoea brought on by my painkillers, I have realised that physically, I am very restricted to what I can do. If I had thought myself stiff and limited in movement after my first mastectomy, I realise I am now much worse. Occurring right under your armpit, a sentinel lymph node dissection is both constraining and painful. Combined with the second mastectomy, the still protruding drains and I cannot lift my arms, twist my body and I'm not even going to attempt my yoga stretches. The only exercise I can try to do, in between downpours, is walk.

With little to do and only my health and rehabilitation to think about, I find myself often browsing the internet trying to understand more about what this diagnosis means, what best I can do to contribute to my treatment. I've accepted without question that I am going to follow the traditional path of chemotherapy and if required, radiation, my diagnosis is serious enough that I would be unwise not to, but is there more I can do? Are there alternative therapies I can explore? I was brought up in Mullumbimby, a town renowned for its alternative lifestyle, its fascination with bucking the trend. I am used to questioning the conventional. The problem is, how does one find out about these alternative options and are they suitable in my instance? Michelle, my old school friend, eschewed chemo and radiation after her own breast cancer diagnosis, in favour of natural therapies. Maybe she can offer suggestions. I know she set up her own *Facebook* page–*Little Red Socks,* and so, along with many other sites, I scroll through it looking for ideas. While I can immediately adopt some of her recommendations, like dry brushing, swapping my deodorant to a natural one and rubbing nourishing oils onto my wounds, others such as intravenous Vitamin C infusions, hypothermia, lymphatic drainage massages, infra-red saunas, meditation, acupuncture, mindfulness and relaxation, I'll have to investigate further.

After a week of negotiations, our offer on that dual key investment unit in Coolangatta is accepted, much to my great delight. It's going to make life so much easier being a 10-minute drive from the hospital where I'll be having all my upcoming treatments. And if truth be told, I love the fact that we will be living in Coolangatta. Brunswick Heads is beautiful, but apart from my bowls, blogs and writing, I have little to do here. Coolangatta, with movie theatres, book clubs and shopping centres, should provide a bit more variety.

It's good to have something positive to focus on, because on Friday, six days after leaving the hospital, I waken feeling unwell. Really horrible. Yesterday, my tight plastic bandage and both drains had been removed in Dr Leong's offices, so if anything, I should be feeling better, free from dressings, tubes and plastic bags, not worse. I've recently discovered podcasts, so feeling achy and hot, I spend most of the morning lying on my bed listening to 'The Thing About Cancer' podcast by the Australian Cancer Council or trying to. I keep dozing off. Paige's incredible hamper had contained a digital thermometer so, feeling a little uneasy, I find it and take my temperature. It's reading 37.9, slightly higher than the normal range of 36.5 - 37.5. It concerns me enough that I phone Dr Leong's rooms. They suggest I call Ward B3, the women's health ward at John Flynn Hospital. I'm fortunate that Lesley is on duty, and she advocates I go to the Emergency Room at John Flynn. While I am loath to partake in a 50-minute drive to the hospital, Darryl is also concerned, and so after grabbing some pyjamas and toiletries, just in case, early afternoon finds us presenting at Emergency. While there is a wait to see a doctor, they do give me an Endone immediately, which helps. They also insert a cannula and take some blood.

It's an interesting wait. I only ever really see an Emergency Room on television; full of hyperactivity and tension, they look riveting. The John Flynn ER is much more sedate. The most concerning case appears to be a young boy who's been bitten by a snake. It's a bit more like television when he presents. At 5.30 pm, three hours after our arrival, my blood work returns.

'There is something brewing,' advises a young doctor with a great Scottish accent, 'we'll just give you a Covid test then bring you through.'

'Will I be staying the night?'

'I would say so.'

Relieved that I had thought to pack an overnight bag, while Darryl retrieves it from the car, I subject myself to this Covid test. It's the most painful one I have had yet and my nostrils are burning, my eyes streaming by the end. Fortunately, it's once again negative, and after bidding Darryl farewell—I'm not sure when I will see him again—I gratefully don my pyjamas and hop into an emergency bed. By 7.30 pm, I'm once again back in Ward B3 looking out at the brightly lit airport with its mesmerising planes landing.

Saturday morning, and while not so long ago it would have been filled with housework, visiting a market or maybe a game of lawn bowls, today I find myself, mask on, being wheeled to radiology for an ultrasound. My blood tests have confirmed an infection and the doctors are trying to determine its exact location. It's obviously come from one of my mastectomy wounds. The fluid building up in each proves that, but which one? This ultrasound should pinpoint its locale, or failing that will determine whether further, more precise, diagnosis via needle aspiration is warranted. This procedure sounds painful and I'm not happy when, a few hours later, the ultrasound confirms the operation will be necessary.

As it's a Saturday, there are no doctors on duty, so it's late afternoon when they eventually find one willing to interrupt their weekend. He comes directly from the beach where he has spent the day with his kids and while they sit in the corridor and wait, he will perform my procedure. I am surprised by this, but extremely grateful.

As expected, it's a horrible experience. The needle feels like a hot angry bee sting as, four times, it pierces my chest, getting samples of fluid. Kate, the pregnant Canadian nurse, helps by diverting my attention with chatter about her upcoming European holiday and tapping me on the leg to distract me each time the needle is inserted. And the lovely doctor whose kids are sitting outside offers comfort with his story about his own mother's recent diagnosis of breast cancer.

'She's not sure what type yet. She's only just been diagnosed. It's been a shock and the whole family is still coming to terms with it.'

While it's unfortunate news and I really feel for him and his mother, it's also strangely reassuring to know that I'm not alone on this scary journey.

The infection that I have caught has really taken hold, so the following day I do little more than lie in bed, trying to make sense of what's on the television. Despite the administration of antibiotics, they don't appear to be working; my chest feels hot, swollen, and painful and I find myself looking forward to the nurses' painkillers, although I am becoming selective. While I love Endone as it gets rid of most of the pain, its effects only last two hours. Plexia lasts longer but makes me sleepy. Paracetamol, for such an easily obtainable drug, is amazing, but must be used with one of the stronger ones. By the end of my stay, I should be an expert!

I've forgotten a hairbrush and some other toiletries, so Lesley goes beyond the call of duty and slips down to the pharmacy for me. While I may visit the pharmacy myself, I'm not feeling well enough, and Covid makes it unwise. I'm incredibly grateful to Lesley, but equally annoyed by my current state of immobility and by the limitations and fear Covid has put on life.

On Monday, I meet the inappropriately named Dr Slack. He's an infectious diseases' doctor, very confident and reassuring. He offers some comfort with his confirmation that they have identified the location and bug causing my infection. With luck, a change in my antibiotics should have me feeling better. I hope so. I've never felt so bad. So low. For the first time since my diagnosis, I've been wondering if fighting it has been worth it. I'm usually a very confident and strong person. To have thoughts like this is very unusual and quite frightening.

The state of my chest when I waken the following morning, doesn't help. Both mastectomy sites are blazing red and full of fluid. The right-hand site has filled so much that thick greenish liquid is oozing down my ribs. Dr Leong is horrified when she visits.

'You're leaking! How long has it been like this? Why didn't anyone inform me? You are going to need draining and, most probably, new drains inserted.'

'New drains.' I wince. 'Do you think so?'

'Yes.'

'How long will they have to stay in?'

'Until the fluid has drained enough to take them out.'

I'm currently on heparin, a blood thinner. It means that I must wait until late afternoon before it's safe enough to perform this new procedure. 4.30 pm sees me back at radiology where I meet Patrick, a lovely, calm, older Indian doctor, Nat the sonographer and Robyn, a very nice nurse. I've often heard the saying, 'it sounds worse than it is', but this operation, to drain the thick, awful fluid that's leaking from me, and reinsert new drains, is much worse than it sounds. One of the most horrible things I have ever had to endure. It's painful but bearable (just), because I'm well drugged, but I can feel them slicing into my skin, squeezing out the revolting fluid and forcing in the new drains. One on each side. The fluid amount is large, and the drains require force to insert. By the time they clean me up, re-bandage me, and wheel me back to my room, it's past dinnertime. The painkillers are wearing off too. Finding out that they have lost my dinner is the final straw. Fed up and in serious pain, I burst into tears. I'm over breast cancer, hospital, the rain, Covid, everything. I just want life to go back to how it used to be.

It takes Lesley bustling in with some lovely colourful bags for my new drains, an Endone and my dinner for me to stop feeling sorry for myself.

Addendum

Equipment to add to your household first aid kit.

A digital thermometer—vital. A cheap one will suffice. Eye mask. Vomit bags (for the car). U shaped pillow. Bicarb of soda. Salt. Heat pack. A good water bottle. Lip balm.

CHAPTER
8

Cancer Stages and Grades

WHILE DR LEONG IS MY breast surgeon, she has recently advised that for the next stage of my treatment, chemotherapy, I'll be in the hands of an oncologist. Today, I meet mine, the aptly named Doc Martin. I love it I have a doctor with this name. Darryl and I are both huge fans of the television series *Doc Martin* starring Martin Clunes, and much of my first book *Bucket Lists and Walking Sticks* describes how, in 2017, we went in search of this Doc while visiting England, and actually found him. My personal Doc Martin visits mid-morning armed with laptop and paperwork and disarms me immediately by informing me that my invasive lobular breast cancer is stage 3.

I'm going to detract once again from my adventure here and explain a little more about a breast cancer diagnosis. I've mentioned some of the more common types of breast cancer - non-invasive (lobular carcinoma in situ, ductal carcinoma in situ), invasive (lobular, ductal, inflammatory), and their subtypes (hormone positive, HER2 positive and triple negative). Remember, mine is invasive (lobular) hormone positive. Now I'll mention staging and grading.

Once the doctors confirm the type of breast cancer, they will assign a stage and grade to determine the severity of the cancer and help in making a treatment plan.

Stages

Put simply, staging means how big a cancer is and whether it has spread.

Stages range from 0 to 4.

Stage 0–These are pre-invasive breast cancer cells which are contained within the breast duct.

Stage 1–Early-stage breast cancer. The cancer is not larger than 2 cm and only in the breast tissue or maybe in lymph nodes close to the breast.

Stage 2–Early-stage breast cancer. The cancer is not larger than 5 cm and is in the breast or lymph nodes or both.

Stage 3–Locally advanced breast cancer. The cancer is larger than 5 cm and will have spread from the breast to the lymph nodes close to the breast and maybe to the skin of the breast or chest wall.

Stage 4–Metastatic breast cancer. Cancer that has spread to other parts of the body. Common places are bones, liver, lungs and brain.

Grading

Grading describes how abnormal a cancer cell appears under a microscope compared to a normal cell. Grading shows how active a cancer cell is and how fast it is likely to be growing.

Grade 1–The cancer cells only look a little different from a normal cell and are usually slow growing.

Grade 2–The cancer cell does not look like a normal cell and is growing faster than a grade 1 cancer cell.

Grade 3–The cancer cell looks very different from a normal cell and is usually fast growing.

While I am a little more educated now, when Doc Martin hit me with the news that my cancer was stage 3, breast cancer stages and grades were something I was very ignorant about. I think I had previously heard of a stage when someone spoke of a cancer diagnosis, but I did not know what this meant. Dr Leong had earlier confirmed the type and subtype of cancer I had; I was so busy coming to terms with this that I had given no thought to what stage I was at, was too oblivious to ask. To have an oncologist come straight and tell me I've skipped stages 1 and 2, and mine is stage 3, is not only an immense shock but also very frightening. Stages only go up to 4. I'm already nearing the top of the class. Suddenly, I'm aware of just how big a fight I have ahead of me.

'The cells are slow growing,' Dr Martin is continuing. 'Which means it's grade 1. I've imputed your data into a program which predicts 15-year survival rates.' As I'm thinking to myself that grade 1 is probably the most positive piece of news I have heard on this cancer adventure so far, Doc Martin hands me a printed sheet.

'I have a 65% chance of living for 15 more years,' I read aloud.

'Yours is less because of your tumour size. Maybe 60 – 61% and only if you follow the treatment plan, which is 16 rounds of chemotherapy over five months, 25 days of radiation, then a hormone blocker for eight years.'

'60%. Ok. Scary, but I'll take it.'

Once Dr Martin has left, I continue reading. Deducting 5% because of the tumour size, with surgery alone, I have only a 34% chance of living until I am 69, 15 more years. Undertake chemotherapy and my odds increase to 45%. Take hormone therapy medication and that's where I get my 60%, 15-year survival rate. Faced with these figures, the decision to have chemotherapy treatment and hormone therapy becomes even more of a straightforward one.

Still reeling from my conversation with Dr Martin and feeling slightly numb, it's fortunate that I'm finally feeling a little better, a little stronger. Dr Slacks' new antibiotics are doing their job. I recommence my walks around the ward and pay more attention to what's going on around me, and to the nursing staff. Lying here, day after day, shift after shift, I notice their idiosyncrasies. Nurse L, the perfect night-time nurse who happily dispenses the painkillers, and no doubt has a slightly easier night than some as we all escape our pain. Nurse J. The newbie. Dependent as we are on their abilities, she makes me nervous as she fumbles with the intravenous drip that feeds me my lifesaving antibiotics. Nurse Karen, the expert at performing heparin injections. Unlike others, when she administers the injection into my stomach, it's painless. And Nurse Carmen, a seasoned professional. No-one else exudes the same calm authority as she does. And as I am becoming familiar with them, so it works the other way. Most of the nurses start to call me by my name and the tea attendant no longer needs to ask me what I would like. She just brings me a lemon tea and a bottle of water each morning and evening.

I've changed from coffee to green or lemon tea, forgone the provided biscuit and now try to drink litres of water a day, for a variety of reasons. Lying here in hospital, with plenty of reflection and study time, giving thought to my diet and lifestyle, noticing how I have been tucking into the morning teas, the nightly desserts, the meaty mains, I've begun to comprehend that if I want to fight this cancer wholeheartedly, beat those dismal 15-year statistics, then I'm going to have to do more than just rely on the medical profession. I am going to have to make some serious lifestyle changes. While I am happy with my physical well-being, my reflections and brief forays into the causes and nourishment of cancer have made me realise my diet leaves a lot to be desired. In particular, sweets. For the past year my craving for, and consumption of, sweet food, has been insane. Never have I eaten so much junk food; chocolate, biscuits, ice-cream, cakes. Analysing this, I can't help but wonder whether this sugar was feeding my cancer. While it's not backed up by all in the medical profession, my investigations have revealed a link between breast cancer and sugar. Reading this, and recognising my strong desire to stay alive, I've decided that food containing sugar is going to have to go. It's the least I can do. Likewise, meat, in particular red meat. Containing strong carcinogens such as n-nitroso compounds and when cooked, other harmful chemicals that have been strongly linked to breast cancer, I've decided to try and eliminate most meat from my diet. I've never been a big meat eater, so this won't be hard. Alcohol, unfortunately, I also discover, is another offender. Affecting my body's ability to absorb folate and, more concerningly, raise my estrogen levels (my hormone positive breast cancer does not need more estrogen),

I am seriously going to have to reduce my alcohol intake. Finally, dairy. I adore dairy. Ice-cream, cream, yoghurt and every type of delicious cheese under the sun. High in saturated fat and linked to increased estrogen levels, dairy, I'm discovering, is not a friend to those diagnosed with breast cancer. Much to my horror, dairy is going to have to go, or at the very least, be reduced. As I said, this time in hospital is allowing me plenty of investigating, questioning, and thinking time. It's made me realise that I can't just rely on others to get me through this. I am also going to have to do absolutely everything I can and if that means strict and unappealing dietary changes, then so be it.

As is sometimes the way of life, it's not long after coming to these conclusions that something happens that really enforces the aptness of my decisions. Dr Leong visits and she brings the pathology results of my second operation.

'The good news is that no cancer was discovered in your right breast,' she tells me.

'Regarding your dissection, I managed to remove seven additional nodes from amongst the scar tissue and unfortunately, six had cancer in them. Some with extra-nodal extension,' (where the tumour has perforated the lymph node capsule).

'So, counting the three you took from my first operation, nine out of ten of my lymph nodes had cancer in them,' I verify.

'Unfortunately, yes.'

It's a shocking outcome and once again, I realise just how serious a battle I have. Foregoing sweets and cheese is going to be the least of my worries.

Day six and I have run out of clean pyjamas. My brother-in-law Jeremy, an anaesthetist here at John Flynn Hospital, manages to obtain some fresh ones for me. Once he has delivered them and left, the NUM (nurse in charge) comes bustling in, asking who that doctor was and I have to sheepishly admit that it was my brother-in-law stretching Covid rules.

This morning, on one of my laps around the ward, I meet Robyn from Ballina. She's wearing the same pyjamas as me, and despite Covid, we stop for a chat. She's in for a lumpectomy, which Dr Google reminds me is surgery to remove the cancer only and spare the breast, usually offered to stage 0 or 1 patients with DCIS or LCIS.

As I walk away from our talk, I can't help feeling envious of what sounds like a far less invasive procedure. This feeling is further compounded late that afternoon when a wardsman arrives to wheel me to the cardiology department for an electrocardiogram, a test to record the electrical activity of my heart. Apparently, it's a requirement before commencing chemotherapy and will ascertain whether my heart is strong enough to withstand the upcoming heavy drugs. Already slightly apprehensive about what chemotherapy will entail, this questioning of my heart doesn't help, although, sitting in cardiology with electrodes attached to my chest, I am reminded of Pauline. Pauline is one of my lawn bowling associates who, two years ago, at the very onset of Covid, was diagnosed with a cancerous tumour wrapped around her windpipe. Pauline had to undergo numerous procedures, including an electrocardiogram before her chemotherapy. While she was initially seen at John Flynn Hospital, subsequent Covid induced border closures between New South Wales and Queensland meant Pauline was forced to relocate to the aging St Vincent's in Lismore for further treatment. Thinking of her provides me with some degree of courage and comfort. If Pauline could get through all of this, then so can I.

In hospital, you're in a completely different world, far removed from normal life. Friday evening and I'm wheeled down to radiology for a brain MRI. Dr Martin wants further details on the meningioma revealed by my earlier PET scan. At this stage, I do not know what a meningioma is and am just happy to be escaping the ward. Despite it being after 7 pm on a wet, Friday night, radiology is buzzing. It's a staff member's birthday, and regardless of Covid, a cake is being shared around and the staff are jovial. Their cheery demeanour is contagious, and the patients relaxed. Except for the dementia patient ahead of me in the MRI machine who keeps struggling to escape the apparatus the moment the operators leave the room. They must keep returning to position him time and time again. If it wasn't so funny, so like a rehearsed comedy sketch, it would be tragic.

On Saturday, Dr Leong tornadoes into my room and whips out my left drain. The action hurts a lot, but it does mean the fight against my infection is being won, the ooze is draining, and I am nearer to going home. It's been nine days now and I'm fed up with hospital. My only contact with the outside world is via my daily breakfasts with Darryl. We *FaceTime* each other over our respective meals and catch up on life. Unable to go anywhere for fear of catching Covid and passing it on to me, Darryl's life has been quiet. The bad weather hasn't helped either.

Finally, on Sunday, Dr Leong gives permission for me to leave. The cannula used to inject my antibiotics fell out a few days ago, meaning I'm on oral tablets, able to be taken at home. My chest is looking better. The bandages have been removed and the two long scars, while still very swollen, are a much healthier colour. Prior to my discharge, a nurse removes my second drain. She is gentler than Dr Leong and it doesn't hurt as much.

Addendum

Statistics – Breast cancer is the most commonly diagnosed cancer amongst Australian women. Approximately, 57 Australians are diagnosed every day. The average age of diagnosis is 62. The relative five-year survival rate for breast cancer is 92%. In 2000, there were approx. 136 cases per 100,000 females. In 2023, this number has increased to 150 cases per 100,000 females.

CHAPTER

9

The Flood

IT'S 5 AM THE FOLLOWING morning, Monday, 28 February 2022. I'm asleep on my back, a position I have been forced into and which I find very uncomfortable when the phone rings. It's Davina, Darryl's youngest sister.

'Mullumbimby is flooding. Unlike anything anyone has seen before. I know Emma's just out of hospital and I'm sorry to wake you both, but dad's flat is flooding.'

'What?' mumbles Darryl. Still trying to wake up.

'He's just phoned me. There's water pouring into his flat and it's up to his ankles. The roads between Lismore and Mullumbimby are totally under water or washed away so we can't get to him. Do you think you can?'

'If the roads are flooded from Lismore, then they will also be under between Brunswick and Mullumbimby.' Darryl replies. 'But we'll see what we can do.'

Not much, it turns out. For the first time in history, most of Mullumbimby goes under in this terrible deluge that has been building for the past month. Houses, which have never been flooded before, are now inundated. The house we sold just weeks ago has been affected and Lloyd, Darryl's father's house, is awash. Eventually, appealing for help via *Facebook*, we manage to get Lloyd removed to the local evacuation centre. Just in time, it turns out. Shortly afterwards, our internet and phones go down and we will remain uncontactable for the following few days.

Hemmed in on all sides by unprecedented flood waters, no internet, I find myself struggling and realise how much escaping into social media and cyberspace has been helping me this past month. Scrolling through my *Facebook* and *Instagram* feeds, getting helpful information from various cancer sites or reading just an online book, allows me to forget about my worries, even if only temporarily. For a while, I can ignore my discomfort, my upcoming chemotherapy, what I am missing out on, my concerning fifteen-year survival rate. With the rain still coming and trying to find other methods of distraction, I attempt my yoga stretches for the first time in weeks and am further disheartened when I find just how inflexible I have become. As I discovered shortly after my second operation, the mastectomies have affected my upper body and it's still incredibly difficult to do much with my arms. Night-time doesn't help. Between those night-time terrors I mentioned earlier and menopausal hot flushes, I frequently wake in the early hours, unable to return to sleep. The perfect opportunity for negative thoughts to fill my head. My mind swings from self-pity. Why did this happen to me? Why did it have to be grade 3? To remorse—but what about all those worse off? What about Jo?

Jo is a former neighbour, a bubbly vibrant lady not much older than me, who I have just learnt, is undergoing more tests right now in John Flynn Hospital. Diagnosed with breast cancer 10 years ago, she managed to beat it, or so she had hoped. Her cancer has returned, unfortunately, this time in her brain. To make matters worse, Jo's house has just been flooded and when she leaves hospital, it won't be to the security and comfort of her own home.

My saviour in my struggles and dark thoughts is Darryl. Having gone through a terrible ordeal himself, he understands my pain, my limitations and my mindset completely. Without his unyielding support, his shouldering of all household duties, his total love, it would be so much harder to fight this fight. To ever get back to sleep.

Thankfully, on 3 March 2022, three days later, it's an enormous relief when the internet and our phones return, the rain abates, and we can go for a long walk. Like Mullumbimby, flood waters have also severely affected Brunswick Heads in some parts, and it's devastating, walking the streets, to see the entire contents of household after flooded household, people's cherished belongings, dumped curb side.

Although the rain has gone, the destruction hasn't. Most roads, including the M1, our main highway, are closed because of either flood water or they have been washed away and no longer exist. I am supposed to be meeting with Dr Martin in his rooms at John Flynn Hospital, but the road closures make this impossible. Instead, he has organised a phone consult and at 9 pm that night, he calls.

'Apologies for the time. It's been a long day.'

I don't need any apologies. All I can think is how amazing doctors are.

'How are you? How is the infection?'

'I'm good. Fed up with the weather, but the antibiotics are doing their job. I'm on them for another nine days.'

'Good. I have you scheduled to have a portacath inserted on 14 March, then you'll begin chemotherapy on the 17th. I'll have Dr Anderson's office email you the information regarding your portacath and someone from the cancer clinic will be in touch.'

It feels good to have a date set for my portacath and chemotherapy. Chemo will take my survival rate up at least another 10-11% and I've been keen to get the portacath insertion over and done with. My sixth operation in two years. For those that don't know, a portacath is a small triangular shaped device that is planted under the skin on the chest wall and is used to draw blood and give treatment such as chemotherapy drugs or antibiotics. It will eliminate a nurse having to insert a cannula into an arm vein each visit and, given my history with cannulas, I am relieved to have a port as an option.

With just 11 days before I return to hospital and two weeks before I commence chemo, I have plenty to keep me occupied. I know I will not be able to see a dentist for a while, because chemotherapy will compromise my immune system, so I make an appointment now. My regular dentist has had two feet of water go through her surgery doors, so I book into my sister Michelle's dentist at Tweed Heads.

While some chemo drugs do not cause hair loss, I have been advised that doxorubicin, one of the drugs I will take, does. I am expected to go bald within a few weeks of commencement. To negate fistfuls of hair falling out while I am in the shower or sleeping, I book in to see Rachel, my hairdresser who cuts it short.

'I don't want it shaved just yet. That will be too much,' I tell her.

'You look like Annie Lennox' she cries after the event.

'I never liked Annie Lennox's look.' I growl.

Where my breasts used to be, fluid has been pooling. Called seromas, they make my chest feel tight and sore and the stitches extending under my armpits feel like deep cuts. To alleviate the pain, I buy a heat pack and find it really helps.

I am continuing with the exercises the physio gave me whilst in hospital and as the days progress, find that despite the stitches and pain, I can do a little more. I even start going for longer walks.

Scrolling through the *Little Red Socks* feed one day, I learn about Chris Wark. Author of *Chris Beat Cancer*, Chris was diagnosed with stage 3 colon cancer at the age of 26. In his book, he claims he beat cancer through natural therapies and nutrition, in particular juicing. He has a popular podcast and so at nights, Darryl and I forgo television, and listen to him advocating huge leafy green salads and pure juices. So persuasive is he that I order a juicer online. It arrives a few days later.

'Look at the size of it,' I cry. 'Where am I going to put it?'

'Why did you buy one so big?' questions Darryl.

'I didn't realise it was going to be so big. It's going to cost a fortune in vegetables and fruit.'

It does cost a fortune in food and it's so big that the only place I can store it is, inconveniently, on our kitchen bench top. It eventually becomes a real nuisance and when, months later, I learn that juicing isn't necessarily the best way to consume fruit and vegetables, it extracts all the essential fibre, I sell it.

One of the hardest parts of my breast cancer diagnosis, I have learnt, is telling those close to me. I'm normally a healthy, energetic, positive person, so can only assume this is the reason I find it so hard. I don't enjoy admitting weakness. But I accept, with a diagnosis as serious as cancer, that I need to let others know, especially friends and family who live overseas; they deserve to be informed, updated. Additionally, many local friends and family are still not aware of what's going on. Some are bound to see me with my new, hairless look. For these reasons, a week before I am due back in hospital, I make an informative *Facebook* post and am totally inundated with messages of support. While it's an incredibly cathartic exercise, it's also overwhelming and doesn't stop me retreating into myself. Probably because I know I am going to need to be strong, I find myself becoming a lot more self-focused, self-centred even. I increasingly find that I only want to concentrate on myself and my immediate family. Not waste even the slightest bit of energy on others. One morning, during one of my walks, I find myself rudely walking away from someone whose conversation about religion is so exhausting, so irrelevant, that I can't handle it. Whereas once, I may have been polite and heard them out, today, I need my strength and energy for more important things.

On 5 March, an event occurs which underscores these notions of needing to conserve my strength, not waste energy on the immaterial. In the very early hours of the morning, I'm lying awake when a news notification pops up on my phone. It informs me that Shane Warne, age only 52, died yesterday alone and in a strange Thai hotel room. Shane Warne was rich, famous, a supposedly fit ex-cricket legend with legions of fans and friends. Yet none of this could prevent him from dying young and alone. It's a difficult analogy, but it makes me realise how fickle life can be. That I need to do what is best for me.

Knowing I am about to begin chemotherapy and thus will most likely not be up to visiting them for a while, one day both Pierce and Paige return together to Brunswick Heads. Entering the house, they both look so young, healthy and vibrant. So carefree. So nonchalant.

So oblivious. It's true that you don't recognise or appreciate your health, your vitality when you're young. It's something that is just there. Having them around, learning to be a mother with cancer, is informative. While all my mothering instincts come to the fore, to not want to burden them—I want to shield them from all this—I find that my kids won't let me. They want to know everything. And when I fill in the details, it turns out they are more than capable of handling anything I have to tell them. Pierce's response when he learns I will be on hormone-therapy for the next eight years sums it up.

'So, mum. You'll be here for eight more years at least, then?'

Finishing my antibiotics is worrying. The infection had been hard to identify, had delayed my chemotherapy and had been so debilitating that I am terrified it may return. All I can hope is that my own immune system will now do its job.

On the day before I am due back in hospital for my portacath insertion, I visit Dr Taylor, for a last-minute consultation, and my new dentist - Tulea. Tulea, a few days earlier, had performed a quick filling and a wide-mouth x-ray. I'm back today for some preventative tooth sealants. Friendly and knowledgeable about breast cancer from her own mother's diagnosis, I am glad I made the switch from my Mullumbimby dentist. She's even helped me understand lymphoedema.

'Mum had 15 lymph nodes taken out during her mastectomy which, a short time later, caused her lymphoedema. Her lymph fluid could not flow through her arm and so blocked up, causing her arm to swell. It's a permanent condition. If you find your arm even slightly tingling or beginning to swell, get it checked out.'

As I depart the surgery, Tulea offers one last piece of advice.

'Mum found lymphatic drainage massages really beneficial. You might want to investigate them.'

Addendum

Dentist - The last thing you want when going through all of this is problems with your teeth. You may not be able to visit one when undergoing chemotherapy. As soon as practicable following diagnosis, visit your dentist. Explain your situation and let them guide you.

CHAPTER

10

Alternative Cancer Treatments

TWO DAYS BEFORE I AM due to commence chemotherapy, I once again return to John Flynn Hospital, this time for my portacath insertion. Although it requires a general anaesthetic and I'm required to go through the familiar rigmarole; Covid test, weigh-in, stockings, theatre, it's a quick operation. Five hours after arrival, I have been discharged, have had catch-up consults with both Dr Leong and Dr Martin, and have met mum for a beverage in the John Flynn café. She's at the hospital for a heart check-up. Diagnosed with COPD (chronic obstructive pulmonary disease) late last year, she hasn't been feeling well.

'My lifestyle has finally caught up with me,' she wheezes. 'Forty years of smoking, drinking and living well.'

'What did your heart specialist say?'

'That my heart beats 25,000 times more in 24 hours than it should. That the right ventricle is shot. My valves are all leaking and I'm living on my reserves.'

'That doesn't sound good. What are you going to do?'

'Go home and have a glass of wine. He also said I should enjoy myself.'

Although the portacath insertion was a simple procedure, the aftereffects are not quite so easy. My shoulder feels like it's been slammed by a kickboxer and when I unbutton my shirt to look at the result, it looks as if he was wearing large leather boots. Dr Anderson doesn't stitch his wounds, rather he uses glue to seal the cut. He's been liberal with the liquid and glue is splashed generously on the left side of my chest, just under my collarbone. Under the clear glue, I can see a fair amount of congealing blood. As I said, leather boots. Although, I do find a positive in all of this. My fresh wound and the pain that comes with it, has taken my mind off my breast scars. In comparison, they are feeling great, and it looks as if the swelling may even be lessening.

With my portacath now inserted, vital for my upcoming chemotherapy, I check to ensure I have everything else I may need. For some months now, via my *Women's Cancer Support - GC* group, I have been hearing about cold capping for your hair, hands, and feet. Apparently, you can put a special cold cap on your head to prevent hair loss, or special gloves and socks on your hands and feet to prevent chemo induced neuropathy (nerve damage that can cause lifelong numbness or tingling in your hands, fingers, toes and feet). While I am not interested in the cold cap for my hair, the procedure sounds complicated and time consuming and I have already cut my hair; I am very interested in preventing nerve damage to my extremities. These gloves and socks, which contain gel packs I can freeze and reuse each session are freely available to members of this support group. Pierce, fortunately, lives close to their head office and has managed to collect and deliver some to me.

Walk, walk, walk. Must get my daily 10,000 steps. With my upper body once again out of action because of the portacath and unable to perform my yoga stretches, I need something to calm my mind and heal my body, and the answer for me, as always, is walking. Feeling guilty if I miss a day, I find myself, and often, Darryl as well, taking long healing walks around Brunswick Heads. As I walk, I cannot help comparing my hunched physique and slower shuffle with others I see.

'Everyone looks so healthy and fit,' I complain to Darryl. 'You don't realise how lucky you are to have good health until it's gone. I'm so envious of them. And my shoulders. I'm so hunched.'

'That will get better with time.'

'I hope so. I used to give the kids such a hard time if they hunched. Now, I've got the worst posture of us all.'

Along with my walks, I've continued to listen to Chris Wark's podcasts at night, started to implement healthier eating strategies and delved further into alternative ways of treating cancer. As I have said, I would be crazy to abandon the traditional path of chemotherapy and radiation, but I am discovering more about supplementary choices. I want to add as many of these alternative options alongside what I am currently doing. At the end of the day, I want to be able to say that I did everything I could to fight this.

So, when Chris Wark advocates I eat large green salads and drink healthy vegetable juices laced with turmeric, amla, garlic and ginger, I do. And when certain podcasts suggest I buy Kristi Funk's book and *Facebook* advises I follow Jane McLelland and my *Women's Cancer Support - GC* group, recommend I eat broccoli sprouts, I do. Kristi Funk is a doctor and the author of *Breasts: The Owner's Manual*, a tome full of information and advice on reducing cancer risk, treatment options and optimising outcomes. Another gift from Paige who finds it at a discount book shop, I've only just started reading it but am already excited as to what it may contain.

Discovered whilst perusing *Facebook* cancer sites, Jane McLelland, like Chris, turns out to be another author and a cancer survivor. Creator of *How to Starve Cancer: Without Starving Yourself*, I download it from *Amazon* and spend the days before I begin chemotherapy, reading it. Diagnosed with cervical and then lung cancer over 20 years ago, Jane was given weeks to live. Through exercise, healthy eating, supplements and off-label drugs, Jane created the 'Metro Map' which outlines her protocol on how to starve cancer. Reading her book, I find it confronting and confusing but so full of information, which makes sense that I immediately order some of the suggested supplements, berberine, curcumin, EGCG, omega-3, red yeast rice, from *iHerb*. A doctor can only prescribe her recommended big off-label cancer fighting guns, metformin, doxycycline, atorvastatin and mebendazole, so these will be something I will investigate further after chemo.

Broccoli sprouts, I learn, contain tremendous levels of sulforaphane (100-400 times more than the adult broccoli), a great nutrient that possesses both anti-cancer and anti-inflammatory properties. Tasty to eat and easy to grow, I order some sprouting jars online and look forward to growing, then eating them.

Whilst reading books on cancer and perusing cancer websites is fine, what I really want is someone to talk to, to guide me, to teach me about alternative cancer fighting options. The names of two integrative practitioners living on the Gold Coast keep popping up, and so I contact them both. Dr Binjemain, the first practitioner, is one of the very few doctors in Australia who know about the Jane McLelland 'Metro Map' protocol. I am incredibly fortunate that his practice is not all that far from me and so, shortly before I am due to begin chemo, I contact his office, hoping to meet with him. Unfortunately, he's a very popular doctor, and I am advised that they can only put me on a waitlist for now. The other practitioner is Manuela, a naturopath who specialises in the support and care of cancer patients. Manuela can offer me a 50-minute Zoom consult (face to face is still out of the question because of Covid) which I happily and excitingly attend. The meeting goes well; Manuela is lovely and can prescribe additional supplements such as palmitoylethanolamide (PEA) for inflammation, Metagenics kidney care to help protect my kidneys, and others that I can take during and either side of chemotherapy that will support my body and health. She also promises to send a follow-up report with additional information. While the supplements arrive and are really helpful, it takes a reminder email before I receive the report, and I have to admit that I am slightly disappointed with it. Containing much information that I was already aware of, such as which foods I should eat or avoid, and to ensure I exercise, I had been hoping for a little more. Thankful at least, that I have access to her good supplements, I may turn to her again further down the track. In the meantime, I'll wait to hear from Dr Binjemain.

Addendum

Oncologist – A doctor specially trained in diagnosing and treating cancer; they will create your cancer fighting program, perform physical examinations and organise any relevant (i.e., hormone blocker) prescriptions.

Radiation oncologist – A doctor who specialises in using radiation to fight cancer; they will perform physical examinations, scrutinize your scans, determine the length of your radiation program, work out exactly where you are to be radiated and help with follow up care.

CHAPTER

11

Chemotherapy

CHEMOTHERAPY IS THE USE OF powerful drugs to kill or slow the growth of fast-growing cancer cells. It can be curative, it can be used to reduce symptoms, or it may be given to prolong life. In my case, I am aiming for the former. You may be given a single chemotherapy drug or several. Doc Martin tells me I will receive two—doxorubicin, also known as the Red Devil because of its bright red colour, and paclitaxel. They can deliver it directly to the cancer or, in my case, through the bloodstream systemically.

Thursday, 17 March, St Patrick's Day and I arrive at the John Flynn Cancer Centre to receive the first of four, fortnightly doses of doxorubicin. It's early, only 8.00 am, I'm fully masked, a little nervous, and I have left Darryl sitting in the car for the next three hours. It will be good when our unit has settled, scheduled for the 29th of this month, and he will simply be able to drop me off then return home. In what should be the first of 16 times when you include paclitaxel, I am admitted, receive my patient identification band and led through to the oncology ward. Knowing they will need to access my fresh port, I am dressed in a button down top, and I have my water bottle clutched in my hand. I've been told that it is best to stay well hydrated in order to flush the drugs out more quickly. Integrative therapy has also suggested I fast for 16-24 hours beforehand (fasting can reduce glucose levels in the blood, making it harder for cancer to grow as well as help with side-effects) but I'm not ready to do this yet. Trying to eat healthily combined with my infection induced low appetite has already put a strain on my weight and diet. I'm not ready to amplify it with fasting.

Doxorubicin does not cause peripheral neuropathy, so for these initial visits, my special gloves and socks have been left behind.

'Hi Emma. My name's Mandy. I'm your nurse this morning. As this is your first visit, I'll give you a run through before we begin. I've been here for 26 years, so I'm familiar with everything. I'll also go through the paperwork. There is a lot of it this first visit. First, just jump on these scales, then choose a chair.'

Mandy has led me into one of three large rectangular rooms, each with eight comfortable looking recliners, four on either side facing each other. Heading the room is an enormous set of scales.

'We weigh you each visit. This will allow us to work out the concentration of your drugs. Ok, 57 kilos. Now grab a seat.'

As I select my recliner, I notice the other inhabited ones are occupied by elderly men. There are no women, which surprises me. For some reason, I had envisioned myself receiving my chemotherapy in the company of nattering females. I had thought that we would sit close together, chatting and comparing life stories. To be seated in a room of silent gnarly males, all of them much older than me, not only throws my expectations completely out the window, but is also disappointing. I hadn't realised how much I had been looking forward to gaining chemotherapy insight and strength through female comradery.

'The drugs we give you can cause nausea and an allergic reaction. To avoid this, we also give you an antihistamine, which will help with any nausea and reactions, and steroids for the swelling and fatigue, and to help with your appetite. You might find it difficult to get to sleep on the nights following the steroids,' Mandy continues, handing me a container containing three tablets.

'We will also go through a list of questions each visit, monitoring any side effects and judging how you are feeling.'

Seeing this is my first visit, Mandy doesn't need to ask these specific questions yet; instead she gives me a bit of a rundown on her life story as we wait for the antihistamine and steroids to take effect. It's informative, albeit a little lengthy, and easily fills the time required for the tablets to do their work.

'Ok, you should be ready now. First things first, I'll run a saline solution through followed by the doxorubicin. We'll finish with a saline flush. All up, it will take around two hours. As this is your first time, while the doxorubicin is going through, I will be closely monitoring you for any reactions. I actually won't be taking my eyes off you.'

'What type of reaction?'

'Dizziness, shortness of breath, itching, anxiety, feeling hot, headache, nausea. If you feel any of these, tell me immediately.'

As doxorubicin is an extremely potent drug, considered one of the strongest chemotherapy drugs for breast cancer ever invented, care with its handling is required. It means that Mandy must wear full PPE (personal protective equipment). As she dons her purple plastic gown, gloves and mask, I mention the newness of my port.

'I only had it inserted two days ago. Is it ok to use already? Will it hurt?'

'It is fine to use already. We have patients who receive their port the same day as their first treatment. It may hurt a bit when I press on it this first time. In future, we will give you some patches to put over it a few hours before arrival. They will help numb it.'

Wishing I had heard of these patches earlier, I hold my breath as Mandy presses a disc shaped device containing a small needle against the gory mess that is my port—much like a power cord plugging into a socket. It's surprisingly painless and the saline solution, which will ensure a clear path for the following medication, is soon administered.

'Ok. Time for the doxorubicin. I'll be sitting here for the entire time it goes in. Let me know immediately you feel anything.'

While it's quite a scary feeling sitting there, having a toxic drug pumped into you, waiting to see if something awful happens, it is reassuring to have a nurse on hand. It takes about thirty minutes to fully dispense, and I think we both expel our breath once it's done.

'Great. You did well. Now for the saline, this will push any residual medication through, then a flush to clear anything, and you will be free to go.'

The saline takes a good hour to feed its way through my body and as it does so; I recline my chair, switch on my television, and monitor my surroundings. Some occupants of the other chairs have been replaced and, much to my gratification, a lady nearer my age and wearing a headscarf is now sitting alongside of me. She looks a bit shattered, and I give her a tentative smile.

'Hi.'

'Hi' she returns. 'First visit? I think this will be my last, thank God. I've done four Red Devils and eight Taxol's. I was meant to have twelve Taxol's but the neuropathy in my hands is getting too bad. It looks like I'm going to have to stop.'

As this is the same regime I will be on, her comments are frightening. I don't want to have to finish early, to not receive the full recommended chemotherapy dose, but insightful.

'Yes. This is my first visit. I'm hoping ice gloves and socks will prevent neuropathy. When did your neuropathy start and when did you notice your hair falling out?'

'I wish I had heard about the ice gloves. I found out too late. I think it was after the fifth or sixth round of Taxol that I started to feel some tingling in my hands. Some numbness. My hair started falling out after my second visit. You will be totally bald by your third.'

While I did have Rachel cut my hair short, it's still an inch long.

'I would suggest you shave it completely before it falls out. It'll leave a mess on your pillow, your clothes, in the shower, otherwise. And make sure you use the ice gloves and socks.'

Mulling over her comments, restricted in movement and with little else to do apart from watch television, I pull out my phone. I need cheering up and so browse a few sites looking for button down tops. Myer is currently having an online sale, which does the trick. As I make payment for a cheering pink fluffy cardigan, a staff member wielding a tea-trolley approaches.

'Tea or coffee and a slice of cake?' she asks.

'Could I have a peppermint tea?' I reply. 'And do you have any fruit?'

'Sorry love. Just cake and biscuits. Don't know why we don't have fruit.'

Thinking it poor that a cancer ward in a hospital can only offer processed food, I accept my peppermint tea. I'll bring my own fruit in future.

Three hours after I arrived, it's all over and Darryl has collected me. Sitting in the car on the way home to Brunswick Heads, we both notice that my words are coming out a little thick and slurred, like I've had a few glasses of wine, and I am certainly feeling fragile. By nightfall, after a day of rest, I'm feeling a bit better and that night, despite the steroids, I sleep like the dead.

As part of my treatment while going through this first stage of my chemotherapy routine, the four fortnightly doses of doxorubicin, the following morning I am required to inject myself with a medication called pegfilgrastim, along with taking steroid tablets for two days. The steroids will help bring down inflammation, manage pain and prevent nausea while the pegfilgrastim will help my body make more white blood cells and thus assist in the fight against serious infection. I take the steroids with my daily calcium tablet and breakfast, and later, I remove the pegfilgrastim from the fridge where I stored it since bringing it home from the hospital the day before.

'I've never given myself an injection before.' I mention to Darryl. 'Luckily, it's already preloaded and has a retractable needle for safety.'

'I had to inject myself with warfarin after my accident,' he replies. 'If you like, I can do it for you?'

'No. I want to learn how.'

It takes a bit of courage and a lot of face grimacing, but eventually I grab a handful of belly fat and plug in the syringe.

'Did it hurt?'

'Not really. And it feels good to have done it myself,' I proudly reply.

Addendum

Lymphoedema - Is swelling that occurs in the arm or leg when lymph nodes or vessels that make up the lymphatic system become damaged or blocked. If you have had lymph nodes removed, ensure you find yourself a lymphoedema physio and additionally, book yourself a lymphatic drainage massage.

CHAPTER
12

Lymphatic Drainage Massage

AS MENTIONED PREVIOUSLY, CANCER PATIENTS look for anything and at everything to help them win the fight. Following my Zoom consult with Manuela, I had bought many of the supplements recommended by her to support my body and organs.

Jane McLelland's protocol makes a good argument for starving cancer by blocking the main cancer pathways, its sources of fuel–glucose (sugar), glutamine (an amino acid) and lipids (fatty compounds). So, I had bought some supplements suggested by her.

It means that currently I have in my arsenal, calcium and vitamin D for bone health, loratadine and PEA for inflammation, green tea or EGCG to increase the effectiveness of the chemo drugs (likewise curcumin), magnesium for muscle health, fish oil, vitamin B, coq10 and a few others. I've run the list past Dr Martin and I am also very aware that I need to ensure any supplement I take does not interfere with the chemotherapy drugs or contravene other supplements. To be safe, I will wait at least three days after chemo before taking certain supplements or will eliminate them entirely until chemo is finished. Examples of these contrary medications are the glucose pathway blockers–like berberine, the glutamine pathway blockers–red yeast rice and the lipid pathway blockers–modified citrus pectin and garcinia. My armoury of drugs is huge, expensive and I hope, worth it.

Although Australia is slowly beginning to awaken after Covid; immunisation is now occurring, border closure rules are relaxing, masks are disappearing, people are socialising; our world is still in hibernation. Neither of us can afford to get Covid, nothing can interfere with my treatment and so our universe comprises just the two of us. No entertainment, no visitors, no fun. If we do leave the house, we are fully masked, and a small bottle of hand sanitiser comes with us.

It also means that when my bowling pennants team attest the State finals a few days later, I can't be there. (They lose unfortunately, but that's beside the point.) And Darryl can't do a thing to assist in the repair of Lloyd's house, which sustained damage in the horror flood. He must leave it to his sisters and incredible volunteers who appear at his door to sort out. Our days have become limited to small walks, television, reading, and resting. Which is fortunate, really, because for the week following my treatment, I feel awful. Despite taking anti-nausea tablets, I feel constantly queasy. My chest wounds swell considerably, as do my feet and face. I develop an itchy torso rash and intense hot sweaty flushes keep me awake at night. Doc Martin had mentioned that patients usually put on weight during this period because of the steroids, but I doubt this will be the case with me. Everything I eat is either flavourless or tastes appalling. Chris Wark's suggested juices and salads look and taste disgusting (and are something I eventually do away with entirely). Food, something I used to adore, has become something to endure rather than appreciate. Even simple water takes on a ghastly metallic taste and I can only tolerate it if I lace it with lemon juice. Thankfully, by about day six, things begin to settle down. While water and some food still taste bad and I'm always slightly nauseous, my energy levels start to improve and the swelling in my chest, feet and face subsides. My chest still feels tight and uncomfortable, but less so. I suspect tight and uncomfortable will be normal for another year or so. It's fortunate that doxorubicin is administered fortnightly, allowing me time to recover between doses, and it's fortunate timing with my dates, because this week, my week off, contains some auspicious events.

The first event, on 24 March, is my birthday. I love having a birthday. I never seem to mind turning another year older. I just look forward to being spoilt or spoiling myself. I can even, usually, string the celebration out and turn my birthday into a weeklong event. This year, the year I turn 55, though we can't meet up with anyone, go anywhere or do anything much, I am determined to still enjoy the day. It starts off well with the arrival of a huge stunning bunch of flowers from my sister-in-law Petria and her husband Dave and progresses with the delivery of a small healthy carrot cake from neighbours Dave and Kay and a gorgeous, scented candle from Paige. A package turns up from Michelle, containing a handmade ceramic mug depicting a woman's chest and while I'm not too sure about this cup and its protruding knockers, it's the thought that counts. Patma, aware that I will need button down tops for chemotherapy, has given me a thick Italian yarn cardigan, the quality of which I could never afford myself, and Darryl has organised (with a little prompting), a lymphatic drainage massage.

Following my conversation with my dentist Tulea, I've been doing a bit of investigating into this type of massage and I have been hearing a lot of great things. The *Women's Cancer Support - GC* group, in particular, promotes their benefits and thoroughly recommends one of their patrons, Sarah Paxford, an occupational therapist and lymphatic drainage specialist. Unlike a normal relaxation or deep-tissue massage, a lymphatic drainage massage involves gentle manipulation and light skin stretching to promote the movement of lymph fluid around the body. The tightness I have been feeling in my chest area and left armpit results from lymph fluid collecting. Whereas once the lymph nodes would help release this fluid back into the bloodstream, my nodes have been removed, thus assistance is required. Failure to prevent the accumulation of lymph fluid could cause lymphoedema (localised swelling). Done properly, it will help with my blood circulation, immune function and, most important to me, chest swelling. Sarah's business operates out of Currumbin, so that afternoon, both of us fully masked and while Darryl waits in the car, I have my first session with Aranka, one of Sarah's therapists. A specialist in dealing with cancer patients, Aranka has no problem with touching and massaging my scars, and at the end of the 90 minutes, having also had white light therapy, I leave with my chest feeling the best it has done in months.

The second event is the purchase of our new property in Coolangatta. Necessitating a visit to the bank on the 27 March to organise payment; a fraught affair following our solicitors' advice to double then triple-check account transfer details to avoid scammers; it's with immense relief and excitement that we obtain our apartment swipe cards on the 29th.

Containing a partially furnished studio we will rent out once we have revamped it and a fully furnished one-bedroom apartment that we move into that afternoon and for the time-being, will be for our personal use, it's going to make life so much easier and enjoyable. To cement a very happy occasion, my sister Michelle, and Darryl's sister Petria, now both close neighbours, have also delivered huge containers of fresh home-cooked food.

With my second chemotherapy session approaching and knowing now how awful I am going to feel for at least a week afterwards, the following few days are spent in preparation. We haven't yet settled into our unit properly and so during this time, cupboards are filled, the building and surrounds are explored, bearings obtained. A few days before each chemo session, I am required to have a blood test to check my liver, kidneys and red and white blood cell levels. Whereas in Brunswick Heads, I would have to drive elsewhere for this, here in Coolangatta, I find four pathologists within a 10-minute walking radius.

Requiring internet to supplement that provided by our apartment building, an Optus outlet across the road provides a modem that can be moved between our two properties, and a nearby appliance outlet provides us with a water purifier. While we have been talking about obtaining a water purifier for many years, my diagnosis has provided the excuse to actually purchase one. Australia's water supply is definitely superior to many other countries, but it still contains chlorine, fluoride, plastic waste toxins, soil residue and other contaminants. Now, being much more aware and concerned by what goes into my body, I think this an essential purchase. It also greatly improves the taste and smell of our drinking water, although I need to continue adding lemon juice.

Addendum

You're going through an incredibly stressful time, you may want to investigate –

Mindfulness – being fully present in the moment and not be overwhelmed by what's going on around you.

Tapping – tapping acupuncture points to relieve stress and anxiety.

Meditation – the practice of using a technique such as mindfulness.

CHAPTER
13

The Aftereffects

———— ∞ ————

MY SECOND CHEMO SESSION AND this time it's an easy 10-minute drive, after which Darryl can return home to wait. Driving myself to my sessions is not recommended because of the debilitating effects of the drugs. This time, my nurse is Erika and I find her friendly, knowledgeable, and fun. As she first questions me on my side-effects, then closely monitors the administration of the doxorubicin, she chats away.

'How's the hair loss?'

'Not too bad at the moment.'

'Be prepared. I would expect it to start falling out after this visit. How did you go with your injection of pegfilgrastim?'

'Strange having to inject myself, but I did it.'

'Good girl. How's your mouth? You know chemo can damage the healthy cells in your mouth and cause sores or ulcers?

'It is sore but I'm gargling and washing it out constantly with bicarb of soda and salt. I make up a cup each morning and use it constantly throughout the day and night.'

'That's great. I'll have to tell some of my other patients. Do you have a good support network?'

'It's hard at the moment with Covid. I can't really see friends or family, but my husband is fantastic. I wouldn't be able to do it without him. I'm still trying to work it all out.'

'Have you got a Breast Care nurse?'

'I have Lesley, but she only works one day a week in breast care. The rest of her time is spent on the ward. There don't appear to be any McGrath nurses on the Gold Coast.'

'There aren't. It's a real downfall. Have you met our cancer care coordinator Korin? She can probably help you navigate the system a bit more.'

'I did meet her while I was in hospital with my infection. She was great.'

'She is great. I expect she will pop in at some time to see how you are going.'

Eventually, when the Red Devil is fully infused, Emily's chatter ceases, and she moves on to her next patient, a young lad about thirteen or fourteen sitting adjacent to me. He's with his mum and he looks very sick. Frail and pale, his clothes hang from him. But in his hands, like all teenagers, is his phone and it is really heartening, despite his appearance, to see him constantly scrolling. Normally, I hate the way kids never look up from their phones. In this case, I am really glad.

I've forgotten to bring an apple with me, something I had vowed to do on my last visit and so when the tea attendant approaches, I ask again if they have any fruit. Although I am reducing sugar in my diet, fruit, nature's sweetener, is going to be the exception for the time being as it is one of the few things that my stomach is tolerating.

'I'm sorry, love. We still don't, but I have mentioned it to the kitchen. I'm hoping they will do something about it. I have got your peppermint tea, though.'

Although I've forgotten my piece of fruit, I haven't forgotten my bottle of water, constantly sipping from both it and my tea as the saline solution does its job. With all this liquid coursing through my body, I need to use the toilet a few times and still hooked up to my drug dispenser, it's interesting noting the colour of my urine. On the first occasion, it's a bright red, the colour of the Red Devil. By the second and third toilet visit, it has paled to pink and will remain this colour for the following twenty-four hours. What is also interesting is that I have been warned that currently, my urine and all other body fluids are extremely toxic. I am to flush the toilet completely after each visit. I am to carefully dispose of tissues and whatnot, and I am to avoid sex and the exchange of any bodily liquids for at least the next three days. Feeling the way I do; this won't be a problem.

This time, following treatment, I know what to do, what to expect, so I act accordingly. I take my steroids, my anti-nausea tablets and administer my injection of pegfilgrastim. Again, the anti-nausea medication doesn't seem to do much, and I feel constantly sick. My chest again swells—the stitches feel tight and uncomfortable, and I feel incredibly fatigued. The only thing I find that helps is walking. The nausea seems to abate a little after a slow walk along the Coolangatta seafront and the tightness doesn't feel so uncomfortable.

I'm loving living in Coolangatta in our little high-rise apartment with its sweeping views of the healing Pacific Ocean, swimming pool and mini-golf circuit, and mentally, I'm coping well. If it takes having to get breast cancer and go through chemotherapy to live in this lovely apartment, then so be it. Even the restrictions brought about by Covid don't feel so bad now that we are living here. While the rest of the world is throwing away their masks, we still cling to ours and our bottles of sanitiser. Important in a high-rise building where the lifts are an easy source of infection spread. Just how much our current life differs from others occurs to me one Saturday night. It's just gone 8 pm and I am lying in bed while Darryl is watching television in the lounge room. As I lie there, the sound of music floats through the window and I realise that others really are returning to pre-pandemic normal. They are back drinking in bars, eating in restaurants, listening to music. Everything that I know is forbidden to us for the time being.

As like last time, days three and four are the worst. It's not so much the nausea and tiredness that is the problem, but the way my chest feels. The left side where I had the axillary node clearance, in particular. It's uncomfortably tight, swollen and painful, not helped by the rash that again develops. Unable to face food nor do much, I find most of my time is spent mutely staring at the television and Darryl is left with keeping the apartment clean, doing the washing, shopping, everything! Thankfully, by day five I start to feel more human, which is lucky because, as predicted by Erika, what was left of my hair has started to fall out. If I tug at it, my hand comes away with a clump of hair in it, and my towel, when I dry myself after my shower, is covered in the stuff.

'My hair also hurts when I lie in bed,' I mention to Darryl. 'I think it may be time to shave it completely.'

We have been preparing for this moment and have borrowed an electric shaver from Dave, Darryl's brother-in-law.

'What do you think?' I ask sometime later.

'You look great,' Darryl exclaims. 'No hair suits you. You have a nice-shaped head. No strange lumps or funny bumps.'

When travelling through Europe a few years ago, we had discovered that couples in many of the Central European countries, Germany, and Scandinavia, slept with twin doonas rather than share one. With our body temperatures completely different, I am a cold fish whilst Darryl runs really hot; I had found this dual doona concept a great idea and while we hadn't adopted the practice on our return to Australia, I am thinking it may be good to do so now. My nights have been constantly interrupted by menopausal hot flushes, exacerbated by the chemotherapy, and a parched mouth, another chemo symptom. I'm finding it not uncommon to be waking nine, ten or eleven plus times a night, boiling hot with a raging need to moisten my throat. Darryl's never been keen on the idea of separate doonas, but eventually, tired of fighting for his half of our covers, concedes. Day six following chemo, keen to get out, carefully masked, and with my energy levels partially replete, I manage to find some single doonas and nice linen covers at a nearby shopping centre, and while my sleeping problems still exist, having my own bedcover, does help.

Something else that will help with my sleep, I discover around this time, is melatonin, a hormone produced in the brain that controls the body's day and night cycles. Many of the *Facebook* cancer groups I am following mention using melatonin supplements either as a cancer fighting agent, a treatment for chemo side effects, such as low platelet counts, or as a sleep aid. Sounding exactly what I need, I order some from *iHerb* at a price much cheaper than I can find in Australia and when it arrives, can't believe the difference it makes to my nights. From nine or more nightly interruptions, I go to six or less and the times in between I awaken, are welcome black voids.

> **Addendum**
>
> Head and Hair - Chemotherapy attacks fast growing cells which includes your hair. This means you are probably going to lose it, so be prepared. Sleeping on a bald head hurts. Make sure you have a soft beanie handy. Learn to tie a chic headscarf. Investigate in a good wig or a fancy cap/hat.

CHAPTER
14

Facing my Mortality

———— ⤬ ————

IT'S THE THURSDAY BEFORE EASTER and time for my third dose of doxorubicin. Now completely bald, I've donned a white cap that I recently bought online and to cancel any macho look that the baldness may have given me, I'm wearing long dangly earrings, lipstick, and that cheering pink fluffy cardigan I bought online during my first chemotherapy treatment. My nurse is again Erika who, after complementing me on my appearance, berates me on my weight.

'55 kilos. You're not meant to be losing weight.'

'I just can't stomach anything,' I reply. 'I'm always feeling nauseous. The tablets don't work.'

'I'll see if Dr Martin can prescribe an alternative anti-nausea tablet. A different one may do the trick.'

I've just started receiving today's dose of the Red Devil when Doc Martin approaches.

'I've written you a prescription for Stemetil for your nausea. We'll see if that helps. We'll also have to keep an eye on your brain tumour and the mass on your sternum. The results of last month's brain MRI show that the tumour hasn't changed but we will still need to monitor it. Once chemotherapy is finished and before radiation starts, I'll send you for another brain MRI and chest CT scan.'

'Brain tumour,' I croak. 'You mean the meningioma?' I still haven't twigged as to what a meningioma actually is and am only now realising that they are brain tumours. Usually benign, problems arise if they grow, compressing the brain or spinal cord.

'Yes. It's a benign brain tumour, but it's close to your optic nerve so we will need to keep an eye on it to ensure it's not getting any bigger. I'm pretty confident the mass in your chest is nothing of concern, but because the sternum is a common area for breast cancer metastasis, we'll need to keep a close eye on it as well.'

Unaware just how much his words have confounded me, Dr Martin continues, 'your blood work is fine. Your white cell count and platelet levels are low, but not low enough to discontinue treatment.'

A few days before I attend each chemotherapy session, I must undergo a complete blood count (CBC). Dr Martin has previously given me what is called a Rule 3 card (a bar-coded pass that is covered by Medicare and identifies which pathology tests I require), which I present to the phlebotomist (person who takes blood). It is the results of this CBC test that determines how treatment is affecting my body; whether treatment needs to be delayed or whether my dosage needs to be reduced. While a low white blood cell count leaves me more open to infection, a low red blood cell count more open to fatigue from anaemia, and a low platelet count reduces the ability of my blood to clot, thankfully, my levels are hovering within a manageable range.

Apart from Dr Martin's shattering brain tumour news, the rest of this chemo session passes uneventfully. The other patients are primarily aging men who can't offer me any advice. The tea-lady still can't offer me any fruit and I am happy to be nearing the end of the doxorubicin stage of my chemotherapy.

When Darryl picks me up mid-morning, he has Paige in the car with him. She has travelled down from Brisbane by train to celebrate Easter with us. To prepare for her visit, she has been isolating for the past four days and if she has had to go out, has worn a mask. This morning before catching her train, she took a Covid test. People have no idea the extent Covid is impacting on the lives of people with compromised immune systems and what they and family members have to do.

It's the first time Paige has seen our new living quarters, and she is suitably impressed. More so because she will stay in the separate studio so will have her own kitchen and bathroom. She is also a huge fan of home improvement programs, so when she sees that this studio requires modernising, she's even happier.

'It will look great with a fresh white paint job, new taps and shower rose. Don't change the mirrors. I can just repaint the frames when you're ready. Some new furniture, a new television and put in a king size bed. It'll look great. And look. I've written all my suggestions on this piece of paper.'

Once again, post chemotherapy follows the same cycle. The following four to five days, I feel like I have run a marathon after being manhandled by an angry bear. My body aches, I'm bone-tired, my chest scars swell and tighten, and I feel sick. Fortunately, not as sick as usual as the new anti-nausea tablets prescribed by Doc Martin work much better. The itchy rash over my torso area reappears. Hopefully, it will disappear for good when I begin my next chemo drug paclitaxel, and this time, I also develop a persistent annoying cough.

I've been very vigilant about my mouth-wash routine, every morning making up a fresh cup of water, bicarb of soda and salt, then gargling with it throughout the day and night. So far, I have avoided any of the mouth ulcers and sore throat commonly associated with chemotherapy and I am putting it down to my constant gargling, day, and especially when I wake during the night.

Unlike previous years where Easter was celebrated with lots of food, alcohol, chocolate and hot cross buns, this year, because of our change in diet, is different. Alcohol, which I now know can increase estrogen levels (cancer fuel) is out of the question. I couldn't tolerate it, anyway. Chocolate, full of high-fat dairy and sugars, is taboo, and the high in carbohydrates (sugar), Easter buns have been replaced by a low GI, high in fibre alternative. As we enjoy Paige's company, go for slow walks around Coolangatta and I recover from my latest bout of chemotherapy, we all acknowledge that it's not the food, the chocolate, the drinking, that makes Easter, but rather the company. Having both Darryl and Paige around has helped enormously with my wellbeing.

Something else that has been helping with my wellbeing during this time is the frequent messages of support I have been receiving from friends and family, in particular, my Aunt Charlotte and her husband Derek, who reside in England. Made familiar to readers of my books, it was in their house we stayed during our recent travels. Interestingly, both Charlotte and Derek lost their former spouses to cancer, and as a consequence, both are very familiar with the whole cancer rigmarole; chemotherapy, and all. Because they understand this cancer journey so well, they, more than most, know exactly how to provide comfort to someone currently travelling it. For example, each fortnight, at the precise time I am undertaking my chemotherapy, they light a candle and send me a photo or a small video of this flame burning brightly. Because they live on the opposite side of the world, deliberate thought has to go into when exactly they light this candle and send this message. While it's easy to strike a match and ignite a blaze, Charlotte and Derek, by timing it perfectly with my chemo, by sending me pictures of it burning, have managed to turn a simple act into something incredible. Something that infuses me with pleasure and comfort while providing understanding and encouragement.

For the first time since we purchased our unit over three weeks ago, we return to Brunswick Heads for a night. While I love our house, love having the space that it provides, I'm instantly aware on entering that currently, our smaller, well insulated Coolangatta abode is much more appropriate. It's much warmer, easier to keep clean and requires virtually no maintenance. Returning to Brunswick Heads after a three-week hiatus also confirms how stifled I feel here compared to Coolangatta, which can offer me so much more. Our relationship is based on honesty and the sharing of mindsets therefore, it's a hard conversation I have with Darryl who can't fault Brunswick and wouldn't want to move anywhere else permanently.

'Brunswick Heads is beautiful, but it's really just a very small seaside town full of cafes and dress shops. We've lived in small towns for the past thirty years; I really want to try somewhere that can offer more.' I try to explain. 'I can't do much now, but later, after treatment, I want access to public transport, movie theatres, airports and shops. I would like more opportunities to bowl, to volunteer, to attend classes. To be closer to the kids.'

'I understand, but you could find more to do in Brunswick Heads if you wanted.'

'I could, but these are the things I want to do. Having cancer, not knowing if I am going to be alive in four, five or ten-years' time, has made me think about what it is I want to do. Made me realise that I need to live my life now. That if I want to do something, I have to do it now or make plans to do it soon. As they say, we only get one life and I've got to make the most of mine before I die.'

I'm in tears by the end of my outburst and Darryl nearly is. Cancer has stripped our lives back to the basics, forced me to acknowledge what I want to do with what's left of my life and created an impasse between us. Should we stay in Brunswick Heads where Darryl is happy and if I should die, where he would live? Or should we sell up and move to where I'll be happy?

'Let's finish renovating the studio, give it to Mantra to manage or rent it out privately, then reassess.' Darryl suggests. 'For the time being, we can afford to keep our one-bedroom flat for ourselves, so we have the best of both, Brunswick and Coolangatta. If the rent on the studio is good enough, maybe we can continue to live between the two.'

It's been a tough conversation with a satisfactory outcome for the time being, and it's voiced a subject that remerges a few days later when I meet my sister Michelle for a walk along the Coolangatta foreshore. I've been too wrapped up in appointments, operations and treatment to reflect on my diagnosis entirely, but that's now changed. I'm fully grasping that a stage 3 diagnosis along with multiple large tumours and extensive lymph node involvement means I really could die.

'What I am most worried about,' I reveal to Michelle once I have caught her up on my full medical situation, brain tumour and all, 'is the kids. I need to know that you will always be there for them, especially Paige. Pierce will have his gorgeous partner Bec, but Paige, she needs to have a female influence in her life.'

'I'll always be there for them,' she promises, 'and you don't have to worry about Paige having a female influence in her life. I'm sure all three of Darryl's sisters will always be there for her.'

Addendum

Cold Socks and Gloves - Socks and gloves that contain a pocket into which a frozen gel insert can be placed. Imperative if you are having any of the Taxol chemotherapies. Enquire with your chosen support group.

CHAPTER

15

Talking about Metastasis

IT IS 28 APRIL, THREE months since my first mastectomy operation and the date of my last Red Devil. I've been feeling good for the past few days. My flexibility is improving. I haven't been as nauseous, and I have had a little more energy. For someone who has been active their entire life, finding themselves bone weary and confined to the couch or bed has been one of the hardest things to come to terms with. My brain, completely addled by the chemo, is even perking up. Probably becoming a little peeved at the drugs my entire body has been subjected to, it's starting to fight back, to think about fresh adventures, future travel, Egypt, Turkey, Israel. It's starting to cogitate about my new book, suggesting ideas, titles and chapter content and it's remembering that I have a blog site and maybe I should pay it some attention.

What hasn't been so good is my scalp. No-one ever told me that a bald head could be painful. That it is better to wear a beanie to bed each night to prevent my pillow painfully rubbing against my hairless head. The top coarse layer of skin on my hands and feet has also vanished, leaving lovely smooth skin in its stead. Lovely to have and feel but a real problem in the shower where my traction-less feet dangerously slip or when I go to grab something heavy, and it slides through my hands. My rash covered torso hasn't been feeling that great either. Similar to small pimples, my trunk is covered in the painful, itchy lumps and I find myself constantly scratching. Despite being able to flex a little more, my chest, under my arms and the area near my shoulder blades still feel numb, tight and uncomfortable. A little like I have on the tightest, most uncomfortable bra ever invented.

To celebrate getting through this first chemotherapy cycle, I have promised myself another lymphatic drainage massage, this time a full body one. I'm looking forward to it help ease my symptoms.

Knowing that this will be my last fortnightly visit, paclitaxel, my next chemotherapy drug, needs to be dispensed weekly, I get weighed, select a chair and settle in. The John Flynn cancer clinic has three bays, each with eight chairs, and I've taken the last vacant one in this bay. All around me are men and women sitting hooked up to machines dispensing lifesaving medication. Surprisingly, only a few are receiving their doses via a port inserted into their chest like I am. The majority today appear to be receiving their treatment via a cannula in their arm. As the doxorubicin courses through my body, one of the other patients gets up to leave. Before departing the building, he strenuously rings a bell located near the door. The ringing of this bell signifies he has finished his treatment. That hopefully, he will never have to step foot in this place again. I look forward to when I can ring that bell, fingers crossed, in thirteen weeks' time.

It's taken four visits, but this time when the tea attendant approaches, she has a smile on her face.

'I've bought you an apple. It's mine from my locker, but next time you're here, I should be able to offer you a choice of fruit. The kitchen is finally going to put fresh fruit on the menu.'

Blown away not only because she is offering me her own apple but because I may have had some influence over the John Flynn menu, I smile back.

'That's incredible. And thank you for your apple. I've forgotten mine again, so it's really appreciated.'

Not long after this encounter, Korin, the Cancer Coordinator, approaches. She has a piece of paper in her hand which she hands to me.

'I've jotted down the name and number of some organisations that may interest you. There is the YWCA Australia. They offer the Encore program. It's a fantastic program specifically designed for women with breast cancer who have experienced a mastectomy, lumpectomy or breast reconstruction. They operate out of Tweed Heads. I've also written the name and number of the breast care nurse at Tweed Hospital. She only works a few days a week and is busy, but she may be able to see and assist you. Unfortunately, there are no McGrath nurses on the Gold Coast. I've also included the number for the physiotherapy department at Tweed Hospital. They run a free program aimed at helping ladies avoid or live with lymphoedema. I'm sure they could be of benefit to you. For fun, I've also included details on the Look Good Feel Better program. It's a free national program designed to help cancer patients look good and feel better.'

My last caller is Doc Martin. He checks in each session and along with confirming that my blood levels are remaining stable, today he again reiterates the need for a brain MRI and a chest CT scan.

'But not until you have completed this next round of chemotherapy. The paclitaxel.'

'When I get the CT scan of my sternum, could it also check my lungs for metastasis?' I question.

Metastasis is when your cancer has spread from its original site to another part of the body. It usually means that your cancer is now incurable, but it can still be slowed, and symptoms reduced. It is feared by all cancer patients, especially those diagnosed stage 3, as stage 4, the next stage, means you have lost all hope of beating cancer.

'We'll look at that closer to the date,' he replies. 'I don't think it beneficial to go looking for new cancers. MRIs and CT scans already do enough to your body. I don't advocate subjecting patients to more and probably unnecessary tests.'

Maybe because it's had the absolute maximum amount of doxorubicin recommended, but this time my body takes much longer to recover. Nine days after treatment, I am still feeling nauseous, the smell of food makes me gag and my weight has dropped to 53 kilos. My annoying cough is still with me, my torso is still tight and the lethargy, lethal. Acknowledging how bad I feel, I am in absolute awe of those younger women with children who are more and more frequently being diagnosed with breast cancer and having to go through this. I am finding it hard to look after myself without the added burden of small children to worry about. Again, I am incredibly glad and grateful for Darryl. During these times where I can do very little, he uncomplainingly does everything. He cleans, he vacuums, he washes and hangs laundry; he dusts and then at night, he presents me with an incredible and healthy dinner.

Waking on day 10, I am exceedingly happy to find that I feel a little better. With my new paclitaxel regime soon to start, I am hoping that the past few days were rock bottom, that the effects of the drugs will never be as bad.

Having endured the Red Devils and, as promised to myself, one morning Darryl drives me to Currumbin for my 90-minute full body lymphatic drainage massage. I'm again fully masked, as is Aranka, my masseuse. Focusing on the lymphatic system, this gentle form of massage, encourages the movement of lymph fluid and drainage of the lymph nodes. Aranka is an incredible therapist, and I can actually feel my tightness easing, the fluid draining, as she slowly works her way around my body. By the end of my session, she has not only helped me to relax completely, but she has reminded me of the benefits of deep breathing, 'it will help with any stress and anxiety you may be experiencing,' and pointed out that my scalp is dry. 'It's a common side effect of chemotherapy. Just remember to treat it to some oil.'

It's Mother's Day this Sunday, but I have told everyone that I am postponing it until at least October, five months away. We can't go anywhere or see anyone, so it feels better to leave the celebrations until we can. I'm regretful that I can't spend time with my own mother, who is fighting her own health issues, but she waves my concerns aside.

'No-one is really in the mood for celebrating anyway,' she tells me. 'I'm happy to leave it until later in the year. In the meantime, I have made you some more food.'

Mum has always been a great cook. Hailing from a large Kiwi family, food and plenty of it, has always been important. Now that we are residing in Coolangatta, just around the corner from her, she has made it her mission, especially since my weight loss, to fatten me up. Each week, we receive instructions to collect another batch of walnut burgers, vegetable soups, fritters or whatever else she comes up with.

While food still doesn't hold much appeal to me, we are both incredibly grateful for what she provides.

Addendum

Websites I found useful -

Facebook – The *Women's Cancer Support - GC* group. *Breast Cancer Support Australia - for women. Breast Cancer Integrative Healing. Jane McLelland Off Label Drugs for Cancer. Healing Cancer Study Support Group. Verzenio Support Group. Lobular Breast Cancer. ILC Sisters. Fierce, FLAT, Forward. Littleredsocks.*

Breast Cancer Support Network Australia - bcna.org.au

Pink Lotus - pinklotus.com

CHAPTER

16

Rock Bottom

ADHERING TO THE RULES OF this next stage of my chemotherapy treatment causes another shift in our everyday living. Whereas the first, doxorubicin phase, required fortnightly visits to John Flynn Hospital, paclitaxel requires weekly attendance. It means that I have only six days to recover between sessions and I need to get weekly blood tests. I've taken to visiting just the one nearby pathology clinic for these, and the phlebotomist, Cara, has started to feel like a friend. I've also, on the advice of another patient, started taking more interest in the results of these blood and other tests. From now onward, each time I visit hospital, Doc Martin, Dr Leong, or any other specialist, I will ensure I ask for my own copy of the results.

'I've found it really useful to keep track of all my tests. To have my scanned reports on hand. To monitor my white and red blood cell levels,' Jen tells me. 'To see if they have changed, declined or whatever.'

Jen is someone a little younger than me who I had met during my third dose of paclitaxel. Seated next to me, she had been occupied with her computer, but eventually had pushed it aside and given me a smile.

'What's kept you so busy on your laptop?' I question her.

'Theology. I've gone back to university.'

Not wanting to show my ignorance, I have absolutely no idea what theology is and only learn that it is the study of God when I Google it later, I move on to a less cerebral subject.

'What are you here for?'

'Immunotherapy,' Jen replies. 'But it's a long story.'

It was a long story but also an absorbing one. Before I relay it, I'll just jump in with another breast cancer lesson. In January, during my first consult with Dr Leong, she had offered me the choice of surgery first or chemotherapy. I had elected to have surgery (my mastectomy) first. This order of procedure - chemo *after* surgery is termed *adjuvant* therapy. Adjuvant therapy tries to kill any cancer cells left behind following an operation and to stop the cancer from coming back. If I had chosen to undergo chemotherapy before surgery, it would have been referred to as *neo-adjuvant* treatment, which is treatment before surgery. Neo-adjuvant therapy can be used to try to shrink a tumour resulting in less extensive surgery, to see how a cancer responds to a certain chemotherapy drug, or as the main treatment for many early triple negative patients whose cancers are usually more aggressive and do not contain estrogen, progesterone or human epidermal growth factor 2 receptors that can be fought with alternative methods.

As an aside—having recently learnt the difference between the two options—adjuvant or neo-adjuvant, I'm not sure, if time could be rewound, whether I would have been so keen for Dr Leong to 'cut it out' so quickly. Neo-adjuvant patients, I have realised, have the benefit of seeing if cancer still exists in the tissue removed by surgery after chemo. They may also have the comfort of knowing their cancer has been completely removed or, if not, then they *may* have the choice of more chemo.

Back in 2016, Jen was diagnosed with triple negative breast cancer and underwent neo-adjuvant therapy; chemo, followed by mastectomy, and radiation. Nearly five years went by and because triple negative cancer has a high association of reoccurring within three to five years, (estrogen positive cancers are more associated with reoccurring after 10 years) Jen had thought she was in the clear, augmented by friends congratulating her on beating cancer. So, when a persistent earache sent her first to a doctor, then to an Ear, Nose and Throat (ENT) specialist, she didn't really think much of it. She had beaten cancer and besides, cancer doesn't return in the ear. It had only taken the ENT specialist a quick look down her throat to shatter her hopes. Her breast cancer had returned, metastasised, not to her ear, but to her tonsils.

'No-one had ever heard of breast cancer reoccurring in your tonsils,' she tells me.

Because metastasised cancer cells are cancer cells that have spread from an original site (breast in this case) to another site (tonsils) in the body, they are still deemed breast cancer cells.

In the time since then, Jen's breast cancer has also metastasised to her brain, which she fought with high dose radiation and her bones. Because she still has two young children at home, she is pinning all her hopes on this latest treatment, immunotherapy. Immunotherapy, usually administered intravenously for up to two years, uses substances either made in a laboratory or by the body to help the immune system do a better job.

As Jen relayed her story to me, I could only sit and gaze at her in wonder. For someone who had undergone so much, her attitude was incredible, and she looked amazing. No-one would have been able to tell that she had lost both breasts, that only last year she had undergone radiation to the head and that currently, cancer was playing havoc in her bones.

While paclitaxel, I have discovered, doesn't cause as much destruction in its aftermath that doxorubicin did, it's still pretty damaging and follows a definite cycle. On the Thursday afternoon following that morning's treatment and for most of Friday, I feel like Wonder Woman. Full of energy, strong as an ox, hungry. All aftereffects, no doubt, of the accompanying steroids, I look forward to these days and use them to go for long bracing walks. Saturday, and I come crashing down, more exhausted even than when I was on doxorubicin. Two of the previous (albeit very wet) Saturdays have been spent nearly entirely watching television or reading in bed, something very alien to me. As is my new bedtime. Before cancer, I would never be in bed before 9.30-10.00 pm, post cancer and my new normal bedtime is 7.30 pm. Sunday finds me a little brighter and by Wednesday, I'm ready to start all over again.

Knowing which days I can function, we plan our week accordingly. If we want to return to Brunswick Heads, we'll go on a Friday. If we want to shop for food, we'll do it on a Tuesday or Wednesday, likewise appointments. We are both eligible and due for our fourth Covid booster shots and this year's flu jab. With the convenience of nearby Coolangatta pharmacies, it's easy one Wednesday, my good day, to simply present ourselves and receive them both.

Although I'm not always keen, we do pop back to Brunswick Heads on a semi-regular basis. Darryl has some goldfish, which he keeps in an outdoor pond in our garden, and he feels he is neglecting them if he doesn't talk to them and feed them once in a while. I am not all that enthusiastic about returning, mainly because it's mid-June now, the beginning of winter, and our house in Brunswick is freezing compared to our little unit. While we time our stays for the weekend when my energy levels are at their lowest and I can spend some of my time recuperating in a warm bed, my fatless body still means I am uncomfortably cold.

One reason I do return and not let Darryl go by himself is because of the shops in nearby Mullumbimby. Mullumbimby, ever since the hippies arrived back in the 70s, has always been a place where you could find good vegetarian food. Over the past five years, with the growth of veganism, the further rise in popularity of vegetarianism, the surge in demand for gluten-free, sugar-free, organic, Mullumbimby has flourished. More and more people demanding a healthy eating and living lifestyle are moving here, and more and more shops catering to this demand are opening. Unlike Coolangatta, which consists of a more elderly population raised on a meat and three veg diet, Mullumbimby is full of people wanting wholesome, healthy food. In Mullumbimby, it's much easier to source food to suit our current needs.

The second reason I need to return this way is because Dr Lloyd, my new GP, is here. Taking over my healthcare from Dr Taylor, who was only here on an internship, Dr Lloyd, a partner in the surgery, is proving extremely knowledgeable as well as energetic and fun. Along with the specialists at John Flynn, she's playing an important role in my treatment.

'You're eligible for a Medicare Enhanced Primary Care plan,' she tells me one visit.

'Is that where I can access a physio or something?'

'It's a plan of management that I can write up and will enable you to access services such as physiotherapy or occupational therapy,' she advises.

'You told me your lymphatic drainage masseuse is an occupational therapist. You could use this plan to access her services. It would enable you five visits per year. She would only charge you the difference between her rate and the Medicare rebate.'

Ecstatic to realise I can get five more massages at a cheaper price; I mention the Encore program recommended by Korin.

'Korin has given me this paperwork, the program is for breast cancer patients and incorporates exercises both on land and in the pool, and information sessions,' I tell her. 'I just need you to sign off on it saying I can physically do the pool and land exercises. I don't know if I will attend yet. It's not for another month or so, but I would like to have the completed paperwork just in case.'

While having nothing to do with medical help, something else mentioned to me by Korin had been the Look Good Feel Better national program offered to both men and women living with cancer. Designed to boost self-esteem and assist with your appearance, the reviews I had read had been really appealing. Those who had attended the workshop had not only been given expert advice on the application of make-up and how to wear a wig, a scarf, or how to restyle their hair, but had also left with huge piles of expensive products. Ever one to love things like this, I had put my name on the list to take part in a session; being full of other cancer patients, I knew it would be safe to attend. Unfortunately, because of Covid, each session so far has been cancelled. Another workshop is due to be run in a few weeks' time, this one just down the road from us in Coolangatta. Hopefully this one will still go ahead.

Addendum

Household Things - You may want to organise to have your groceries home delivered for a while. Maybe stock your freezer with some pre-made meals. Don't stress about housework—you have more important things to focus on.

CHAPTER

17

Coffee Helps

⁓

MY ANNOYING COUGH IS STILL a worry, and one Thursday immediately following treatment, Doc Martin sends me for a chest x-ray.

'I don't expect it to be anything,' he advises, 'but we need to check.'

The results of the x-ray don't turn up anything nasty to my whole family's utter relief, as the lungs are a common site for breast cancer metastasis, but I wish I knew what was causing the cough.

'It's not common,' Doc Martin tells me. 'But it is more likely a side effect of your chemotherapy.'

While I cannot fix my cough, five rounds into my current chemo cycle or session nine overall, and I am finally winning the battle against my nausea. While the new tablets have helped, it was reintroducing a daily coffee, in this case an almond latte, into my diet that changed everything. Back in February, I had eliminated my morning coffee in favour of green tea, in particular matcha, a green tea especially high in antioxidants. After some reading, I had lately learnt that past studies linking coffee to breast cancer had been proven false, that coffee could actually play a preventative role. I have always appreciated my daily coffee and while I am only going to limit myself to one a day; I am very happy to become reacquainted with the beverage, not least because it introduces into our lives a practice that continues to this day. Mid-morning, every morning, Darryl and I will head out with our Keep Cups to find somewhere to have this coffee. Sometimes Darryl will bring a coffee made at home, but I never do. With my breast cancer diagnosis, having to face my mortality means I'm not so concerned with skimping on what's best. I'm now determined to enjoy life while I can. Turn a blind eye to the expense. We usually take a stroll along the Coolangatta foreshore, or the Brunswick Heads break-wall in search, meaning we are also getting some exercise. This exercise combined with an almond milk latte is not only the perfect antidote for my upset stomach but also gives our mornings a purpose along with stimulating our brains. It becomes the time that we can reconnect, discuss issues, make plans. The focal point of our day. For years, we had scoffed at those enjoying a regular morning beverage. Now we fully understand. It's over this coffee one morning that a memory pops up on my phone and our conversation turns to the subject of travel.

'Can you believe it's been nearly two and a half years since we returned from our last trip,' I utter in disbelief.

'Covid has made the years disappear,' Darryl replies.

'A few months ago, even a few weeks ago, I thought we would never be able to travel again. I wasn't sure I would even want to. But now, things are changing. I'm feeling a lot more positive about everything. The future. I might even start doing some research.'

'If we can and do, travel again, where would you like to go this time and for how long? I don't want to be away as long as previous.' Darryl interjects.

'Istanbul and Egypt are still on my Bucket List. And Jerusalem. Somehow, if everything goes well, continues as they have been, I need to work out how we can visit all three.'

While it may have been a coincidence, my chemo tolerance may have peaked just when I rediscovered coffee, but this period feels as if it is the turning point in my treatment, the BC (before coffee) to AD (after discovery). BC and I felt continuously sick, weak, lifeless. AD and my appetite is slowly returning, my energy levels are rising slightly (although I'm still in bed by 7.30 - 8.00 pm), my morning stretching is becoming a little more regular, and life is looking a bit better. I'm feeling improved enough that when the *Cooly Rocks On Festival* returns to Coolangatta after a few years Covid hiatus, I find the energy to spend a few hours walking with my mask securely in place, amongst the multitude of hot-rods and custom cars on display. And when Paige returns during Uni break with even more ideas on how to renovate our studio, I am happy to support her and Darryl in their renovating endeavours. I can't do much physically, but I can throw in my opinions and advice and watch as the studio is transformed with modern furniture, fresh paint and a new king-sized bed.

Chemo session number 10 sees me paired again with Mandy, the talkative nurse. Now that I am on paclitaxel, the staff don't need to monitor me as closely and following my weigh-in and side-effect probing, will administer the drug then quickly move on to another patient. Before she moves on, Mandy does make a comment on my hair, which, as usual, is covered by a cap.

'Sometimes hair starts to grow back during paclitaxel, is yours?'

'I think it is,' I grin. 'If you look really closely, I think there may be some fine hairs growing. But I've now noticed that both my eyelashes and eyebrows are disappearing. My eyebrows are tattooed, so that doesn't worry me, but my eyes are starting to look weird with very little lashes. I'm not sure how they are going to look when they have completely gone.'

'Everyone reacts differently, and they will grow back,' she assures me. 'Are you sleeping?'

'A little better now, but that's only because of the melatonin and wearing an eye mask. The hot flashes are still awful. I'm probably waking up six or seven times a night.'

'Unfortunately, I expect they may even worsen once you begin hormone blockers.'

With only five more chemotherapy sessions to go, it's time to start preparing for the next stage of my treatment, radiation therapy—the use of high energy waves or particles to destroy cancer cells. For this, I have been referred to a radiation oncologist operating out of Genesis Care, the private cancer service attached to John Flynn Hospital—a doctor with such a long name that I'll just call her Dr T. So that I am fully organised before the commencement of treatment, I meet with Dr T, one Thursday afternoon following that morning's chemotherapy session. Her offices are located immediately above the chemo clinic, so are easily accessible and it's not long before I am ushered into her rooms. It's a 50-minute consult and during that time, I learn some pertinent information, some good, some not so great.

'Although your cancer is grade 1 in that the cells still look similar to normal breast cancer cells, its spread, that it's in so many lymph nodes, makes it more indicative of a grade 3 cancer,' she tells me.

'Because radiation is an out-patient treatment, private health insurance does not cover it in Australia. Most of it will be covered by Medicare, but there will be an out-of-pocket expense.'

'How much would that be?'

'You need to discuss that with our finance department. They will phone you sometime during the following weeks.' As I ponder the cost of this, Dr T continues.

'Because your cancer occurred in your left breast, the side of the chest where your heart is situated, in order to reduce the radiation dose to the heart you will have to learn the deep inspiration breath hold (DIBH). This brochure explains the procedure and what practice you should do.' As I quickly scrutinize the pamphlet Dr T has handed me, she hits me with one final piece of news.

'I've noticed that your port has been placed on the left-hand side of your chest. It will have to be removed before commencing radiation.'

It goes without saying that I am pretty dazed by the time I leave the building. In one intense conversation, I have learnt that my cancer may be even worse than I had thought, that I might have a large bill coming up shortly and that I have to have yet another operation. Ports are normally left in for a few years just in case further treatment is required. It looks as if I'll have mine for just five short months. Although, to be honest, I am not unhappy that my port will be coming out. I haven't complained but actually I hate my port. An obvious lump just beneath my collarbone, it's cumbersome, ugly and very uncomfortable. The glue has not completely gone, it's an infection worry, and I am always painfully bumping it. I'm glad it's going.

Making my way into the chemotherapy clinic for my second last chemo session, I smile wryly to myself under my mask and think how well I've got this routine mastered. Get weighed—I seem to be stabilising at 53 kilos, find a recliner with a good headrest and an interesting view, switch on the television, swallow my two steroids and one antihistamine tablet, pull out my phone and drink bottle, get comfortable. As the nurse robes up then flushes my port, it's time to put on my special ice-shoes and gloves which seem to be working as apart from some sporadic tingling in three toes, I have had no problem with peripheral neuropathy and look likely to complete all sixteen rounds of my treatment. When the tea attendant rolls around, ask for a peppermint tea and an apple, as fruit is now a permanent fixture on the menu. While the paclitaxel is being administered, drink as much fluid as I can, then start flushing it out by going to the toilet. Finally, after the last saline flush, wait to be unhooked from any machine, remove my ice-socks and gloves, put on my shoes, then depart the building.

We are well into winter now and I am again so appreciative that we are living in Coolangatta where the weather is warmer than Brunswick Heads, although it is only a short 40-minute drive away. We have found a regular place to have our morning coffee, the outdoor café attached to the Coolangatta surf club, and we have become regulars, complete with loyalty card. Although I am still fully masked and wear a cap, the staff, Stacy, Travis, Maddy, Jess and Kaitlyn, all recognise me and have taken to calling us by name. A small thing but so uplifting during this time. Along with the warmer climate, I am also appreciating the convenience of having four supermarkets within a short radius. Our new healthy eating regime is more conducive to making daily small purchases of fresh produce rather than one large weekly shop that I used to do. The only problem we are finding with eating mainly a plant-based diet is having to come up with new dishes. Mum's contributions are helping, but most nights tend to find us eating similar things: sweet potato, large green salads, tofu and beans. I'm looking forward to post treatment when I can really put some energy into exploring alternative dishes.

We have had good news regarding our studio. Its revamp is complete, and it is now part of the Mantra pool. We expect to start seeing a return sometime within the following few weeks. I've also some other good news. First, is my hair is definitely starting to grow back. It's very soft, very white and rather fluffy, but it is visible in the mirror. Unlike my eyebrows and lashes, they unfortunately have completely disappeared. Second, I've been accepted into the YWCA Encore program. While I had initially been hesitant to start the program just now as it starts the day after my chemotherapy finishes, the co-ordinator who I spoke to recommended I do it while I can.

'There are rumours that its budget will be pulled in the new year,' she advises. 'Applicants have been dropping, especially in regional areas. It's mentioned that its funds will be redirected towards the homeless and domestic violence.'

The third piece of good news is a double-edged sword. A short while ago, I had been contacted by a Look Good Feel Better facilitator and told that the Tweed Heads' session had been cancelled yet again. Understanding my disappointment, this was my third cancellation, she had mentioned that I might receive a parcel containing some goods in the mail. Yesterday, contrary to my expectations, a parcel had arrived so full of amazing body and face products, I had been completely stunned. Instantly mollified. Researching the items, I found I had received a foundation costing over $250, lipsticks worth $70, a cleanser valued at $65. I had non-toxic moisturisers, vegan body lotions, organic blushes. As I sorted through all the gorgeous items, I realised they were doing or would do, exactly as promised. They would make me look good, and they were certainly making me feel better.

Addendum

Biopsy - A breast biopsy is a procedure that removes tissue or sometimes fluid from a suspicious area of your breast. These samples will be examined under a microscope to see if they contain cancer cells. My biopsy was called a core needle biopsy and was performed using a hollow needle. This is the most common type of breast biopsy. I was able to lie on my back and I found it only mildly painful.

CHAPTER
18

Breast Prosthetics

IT'S THE MORNING OF MY final chemotherapy, 28 July and also, coincidentally, Paige's birthday. She's studying hard at university, so we won't be able to catch up with her and celebrate both events, but not getting together is something everyone has become used to over these past few Covid years. As I take my morning shower in preparation for getting dressed and going to John Flynn, I take a good hard look at myself. My fluffy hair is even more visible now and I'm definitely liking its colour. I had been worried that it would regrow an aging grey, but it's more a vibrant white interspersed with grey. My pubes and leg hair, which had both disappeared when my head hair went, are also regrowing, but there is still no sign of my eyelashes, which is frustrating as eyelashes keep things from blowing into your eyes. At 53 kilos and standing 172 cm tall, I certainly look bony, but like my hair, I don't mind my new body shape. My breast scars are still raw and obvious, but again, I'm not unhappy with their appearance. I have been incredibly vigilant with rubbing either bio-oil or breast balm onto them day and night (something I still do twelve-months later), and I know that my diligence is paying off, they are healing well.

It feels amazing to enter the cancer clinic knowing that this will be my last visit. For some reason, I am allocated two nurses, Erika, who I have had before, and Alison. Time flies with the both of them looking after me and before I know it, I am removing my ice-gloves and socks, ready to depart.

'We have something for you before you leave,' Erika says.

'Yes,' continues Alison. 'One of the local charities donates quilted rugs to be given to those who have gone through chemotherapy. We have a few here. They're gorgeous.'

'Take your pick', says Erika.

They are gorgeous and I happily select a brightly coloured patchwork quilt that's obviously had a lot of work put into it and on which I will now perform my morning yoga stretches.

'I have something for you as well,' I reply, pulling out some copies of my latest book, *Itchy Feet & Bucket Lists*. 'Put them in your staff room.'

'Did you write this?' Alison cries.

'I love travelling,' interrupts Erika. 'I'll love reading this and I know many of the other nurses will as well. Thank you.'

'Yes, thank you,' says Alison. 'They will certainly be read. Now you just have to ring the bell and you're finished.'

Not one to like drawing attention to myself, I find it slightly embarrassing ringing the bell, having people clap and cheer, but knowing exactly what it signifies, I am not going to let embarrassment stop me. I have worked damn hard for this occasion. I've made it through sixteen chemotherapy sessions spanning twenty weeks. Twenty weeks of nausea, fatigue, hair loss, weight loss, constipation, diarrhoea, brain fog, mood swings, plunging blood counts and goodness knows what else. Needless to say, I ring that bell well, then walk out the door.

While it definitely feels like the end of a very big chapter, I'm fully aware there is still a long way to go yet on this cancer fighting adventure and a lot still to do. Tomorrow morning, I will be seeing the lymphoedema physiotherapist at Tweed Heads Hospital before commencing the YWCA Encore program later that afternoon. Next week, it's back to John Flynn Hospital to have my portacath removed and then two weeks after that, I will begin five weeks of radiation. As a reward for dealing with all this, Darryl and I have decided to treat ourselves to an electronic scooter each. We just have to find time to investigate and purchase them.

Some months ago, Korin, John Flynn's cancer care co-ordinator, had given me the name and phone numbers for both the breast care nurse and lymphoedema physiotherapist operating out of Tweed Hospital. While I have not been able to see the breast care nurse, there are too few of them and she has been too busy, I have managed to make an appointment to see Jenny, the physio. Today is my first appointment and to test the strengthening of my body and to celebrate the loosening of my chemotherapy shackles, I walk the 15 minutes it takes to get from our Coolangatta unit to her office.

'The New South Wales government has provided funding to operate a lymphoedema program at various hospitals,' Jenny tells me. 'Whereas once we used to take precise measurements of each arm using a tape measure, to monitor for any swelling, now these technical new machines do all the hard work for us. Although I still like to take your measurements the old way as well.' As I stand on what looks very similar to a large set of upright scales, my hands resting on some metal plates, an iPad-like device computing my results, Jenny continues.

'It's really important that you keep an eye out for swelling. Once you have lymphoedema, it's a lifelong condition. I'm going to give you a compression sleeve. At the slightest sign of swelling, put it on. A sleeve is the best method for the prevention or control of lymphoedema.'

Having come across a few breast cancer survivors with lymphoedema while in hospital, their arm disturbingly swollen, I had realised just how debilitating and awful this side-effect could be. I have no wish to be added to their numbers and so gratefully accept the sleeve Jenny has offered me. I will definitely be donning it if I see any sign of swelling.

Whilst I had been happy to be accepted into the YWCA Encore program, a scheme involving land and pool exercises, it had caused a few dilemmas, the first being what to wear. Having lost both my breasts and some kilos, all my existing swimming costumes are out of the question. The bottoms fall off me, and the tops are useless. You need boobs to stop a swimming top riding up. Someone had suggested I just go topless, but I know that society is not ready yet to accept an exposed scar-covered female chest, even though I have no nipples and am flatter than most men. In the end, I buy a cheap pair of swimmer bottoms from K-mart and use an old rashie for my top. The second problem is whether I will have the stamina to participate, especially so soon after finishing chemo. With only one way to find out, that afternoon I make my way to the Tweed Heads Community Centre where I meet Kim, our facilitator and fellow participants, Nicki, Linda and Di.

Kim is a bubbly curly-haired blond lady and after apologising for the low numbers, this once very popular program is, unfortunately, seeing fewer and fewer applicants, soon has us gently raising our arms, stretching our legs and remembering that once upon a time, doing this wasn't so difficult.

'From next week onwards,' she tells us during a break. 'I'll have a different presenter coming in each session to host a talk on various subjects. I think next week is the Dragon Boat lady or it could be a lady talking about breast prosthesis. If it's her, she'll have some examples you can try on and purchase. I'm not sure if you are aware, but for each breast prosthesis you purchase, every two years, you are eligible for a Medicare rebate of up to $400. So, if you have had two breasts removed, you can get a rebate of $800. For the following weeks, I've also lined up a lymphatic massage specialist, someone selling swimwear for those who have had mastectomies and one or two others. It should be an excellent program. Today, with no speaker, we can just hit the pool a little earlier.'

I had been aware of the Australian Government's rebate program concerning breast prosthesis and had used it to purchase two of the cheaper models (the more expensive ones can go for close to $500 each). While I think it's a great program for those who cannot live without breasts, my prostheses are currently sitting at the bottom of a draw and probably will continue to do so for the rest of their lives. So far, I'm loving being breastless, not having to worry about a bra.

The Encore program has been operating in Australia for over 30 years and was originally developed in the United States by a ballet teacher, Helen Glines Kohut, who had herself gone through breast cancer. Seeing a need to assist others in rebuilding their strength, flexibility and emotional well-being following breast cancer treatment, she had come up with the program we are now undertaking. While not all that keen to jump into the cold pool, I appreciate the quality and focus of Helen's exercises and finish the lesson, feeling not only happy for having managed to complete the session, but for doing something that resembled my old life.

The following few days and it's obvious I have overdone it slightly—commencing an exercise regime so close to chemotherapy. Adding neglected exercise to an exhausted body means all I want to do is recline on the couch. Fortunately, I've just taken advantage of a three-month free trial of *Amazon's Kindle Unlimited* (a subscription program that allows access to millions of online books) which is having a few, happy consequences. The first is, with so much content, so many genres to choose from, it's easy to stay occupied during this enforced lounging time. The second consequence is related to the exact genre I find myself focusing on—travel memoirs. Being a keen reader of this type of book that mentally transports me to countless exciting destinations, it's not long before my ever-itchy feet start twitching once again and I do as I said I would a short time ago over coffee. I pull the computer out and begin to research travel options. It may still be sometime before I'm strong enough to journey again, but just turning on a computer and investigating travel routes signifies to me that, mentally, I have turned a real corner. That I can see light at the end of a very long tunnel. My focus is no longer going to just be about treatment and not dying. I'm not going to let cancer dictate my life. We will travel again.

Addendum

Melatonin Supplements - Melatonin is a hormone naturally produced by the body to regulate the sleep-wake cycle. I wouldn't have been able to function without it. Australians under 55 require a prescription.

CHAPTER

19

Radiation

———⧓———

WEDNESDAY, 3 AUGUST AND ONCE more I'm back at John Flynn Hospital, this time for my portacath removal. With Australia and most of the world now resigned to living with Covid, I may show my negative Covid test completed at home, on check-in. The removal of my portacath is a quick standard operation which goes without a hitch, the only memorable part being the insertion of the anaesthetist's cannula into my arm. It's so incredibly painful that it makes me cry and my last memory before blacking out is him saying, 'I'll hurry and put you under.'

The following week, as I recover from this operation, passes slowly. Perhaps indignant that I have subjected it to so much, my body screams at me. My breast scars throb, my arms and legs ache, I'm totally drained of energy. The only thing that helps is the purchase of two Vsett 8 electric scooters. They cost more than we were expecting, but they are also more durable and powerful. They will easily be able to take us on jaunts of up to 80 kilometres distance. 'Not that I think we will travel that far,' Darryl reassures me.

As mentioned by Dr T during our consult, I'm contacted at this time by the finance department at Genesis Care. If I wish to undergo private radiation therapy with them, as opposed to treatment at a public hospital, they explain, the cost will be $29,000. Medicare will fund $23,000 and they can offer me a discount of $4,400, meaning my out-of-pocket expense will be $1,600.

The closest public hospital to me that offers radiation is the Gold Coast University Hospital, a 40–50-minute drive from Coolangatta through heavily trafficked areas. I will need to attend radiation treatment five days a week for five weeks. It is these factors, along with all the positive reviews I have heard about Genesis Care, that allow me to reply in the affirmative. Yes, I will have radiation treatment with them. In that case, I am told, I will need to attend their offices early next week for a simulation lesson.

The day before I attend this simulation, news channels worldwide are full of Olivia Newton-John's death from breast cancer. It's a real blow hearing this news. If someone with the resources of Olivia Newton-John, founder of the Olivia Newton-John Wellness & Research Centre, a place dedicated to providing cancer sufferers with world leading treatment, hasn't been able to beat breast cancer, then what hope is there for me? Scrolling through the many *Facebook* cancer groups I am now a member of, I realise my feelings are widely shared. We are all feeling a little more vulnerable, a little more disappointed.

One week prior to the real thing, I walk into Genesis Care for my radiation simulation appointment. The staff are all very welcoming and, after completing some paperwork, a nurse explains what is about to happen.

'Today is all about planning and practice. Your radiation team will be carefully mapping out the area of your breast, and because you had lymph nodes test positive for cancer, your underarm area as well, to target exactly where you need treatment. You will have a CT scan that enables the radiation oncologist to see which areas to avoid and which areas to treat. Once they have this information, a template will be made, and marks made on your body. This template and these marks will guide the radiation therapist on future visits. No radiation will be used today. Any questions?'

'I've read that the marks are permanent?'

'They used to be. These days we use heavy-duty stickers. They normally last the course, but it doesn't matter if they do fall off. The template will enable the technician to know exactly where to target treatment.'

'Does it hurt, and will I burn?'

'The radiation therapy itself is painless and only takes around five to ten minutes. You may start to feel uncomfortable as it takes around ten minutes to position you beforehand. After a few weeks, you may notice your chest area reddening. Sometimes the skin may blister. You will be given a sample of Epaderm Cream, which we recommend you apply every session immediately after treatment. It's important that you apply nothing to your chest area before treatment each day. Have you been practicing your deep breathing?'

'I have. I'm a little worried about that. I'm not sure I'll be able to hold each breath for that long.'

'It only needs to be held for 20 seconds. You'll probably find it becomes easier once treatment has begun. Most normally do.'

With those reassuring words, the nurse then hands me a long dressing gown. 'This is yours to keep. Bring it to all future visits,' and directs me to the change room. Here I remove my top, I can keep my pants on, put on the gown, then make my way into the radiation room where everything goes as the nurse had outlined. An hour later, I depart the building, a new green dressing gown and a sample of cream in my bag, three heavy-duty stickers stuck to my chest.

After three cancellations, I've received news that the Look Good Feel Better Tweed Heads workshop is finally going to go ahead the morning of my first radiation session. I've advised them I have already received a goods package in the mail, but they want me to attend anyway, 'Not only can we show you how to use the products but it's a chance to meet others going through the same thing.'

The workshop is being held at Club Tweed, a five-minute walk from me and along the way I purchase today's almond latte. They are still doing wonders for both my stomach and my fatigue. I'm the last to arrive and seating myself, I look around. There appear to be only five other attendees and each, like me, is sitting in front of a mirror with an extensive selection of toiletries, makeup and other beauty paraphernalia alongside. Facilitating are two gorgeous young females with immaculate hair, makeup, and clothing. We will obviously be in expert hands. Before we begin today's session, Kalie, one of the facilitators, directs our attention to a nearby table and advises us to help ourselves to morning tea. I'm still drinking my coffee but thinking it may be nice to have something to eat with it, make my way over to where Kalie is pointing. I find a table groaning under a selection of cakes, muffins and cookies, but not a piece of fruit or healthy item in sight. Returning to my seat, disappointed and empty-handed, I can't help pondering this and wondering if things will ever change. Cancer patients should not be offered food like this. Our bodies are at their lowest and weakest. We need everything we can to make them healthier, stronger. Despite this, the workshop is incredible. There is someone else like me, bald, and we both love trying on various wigs, laughing at the effect and learning how to stylishly tie a headscarf. We have all been given our own foundation, lipstick, blusher, mascara, eyeshadows, cleanser, toner and whatnot and eagerly listen as both Kalie and Jess offer suggestions on how best to apply or use them. At the end of the workshop, we all leave with made-up faces not quite as expertly applied as Kalie and Jess's, but close.

'I don't normally look like this,' is the first thing I say to my radiation technician when I arrive at Genesis Care for my radiation session a few hours later. 'I've just attended a Look Good Feel Better workshop.' I'm bald, barefoot, in my robe, with a full face of make-up and about to be led into one of the two rooms used for radiation therapy. I'm feeling a bit ridiculous. After laughingly assuring me I look great, the technician continues.

'We have two machines for radiation—we call them Yelgun and Northern Rivers. Today, you will use Yelgun, which means you need to wear these goggles. Through them, you will see a thick bar which will rise and fall with your breathing. When we tell you to, take a deep breath and try to get that bar moving upwards as high as possible. Taking a deep breath will move the heart away from the radiation beam.'

Putting on the goggles, I lie back and let the technician and her assistant push, prod and pull me until I am lying exactly where they want. They've used the plastic template made at last week's simulation lesson, and the stickers on my chest, to guide them. While the plastic template used for positioning only, gets removed, a cold, thick silicone mat remains on my torso for protection of my other vital organs. It takes around 10 minutes to complete the important part of the session and I find the deep breathing really hard; I can never quite get that bar to reach the top. It's painless as promised, but I'm feeling disappointed as I rub cream into the radiated area before getting dressed. I'm hoping it will be easier tomorrow.

It's a very early 7.00 am appointment when I return to Genesis Care. Each Friday, we will be given a timetable of the following week's sessions and currently mine, I've noticed, are all between 7 and 8 am. I haven't had to be out the door at this time for months; even chemo was usually later. I don't mind as I've always enjoyed this time of morning when the temperature is lovely, people are exercising and shops, offices and buildings are not yet busy.

This time I am led into Northern Rivers, the alternative treatment room, where I find I do not need to wear goggles. Instead, an iPad shaped screen hangs directly above my face. I have no idea if it's because I don't have something like the goggles pressing against my cheeks or whether it's the machine itself, but this time I find the deep breathing easier, and the session passes smoothly. Glancing at my timetable in order to find tomorrow's session time, I am very relieved to see that my following appointments will also be held in Northern Rivers (in fact, that first session was the only time I ever did use Yelgun).

Genesis Care is a well-oiled organisation, a fact I discover over the following weeks. With close to 90 patients a day to juggle between two machines, I suppose it has to be. While Fridays are the designated day for timetable distribution, Mondays, I learn, are the day for seeing the occupational therapist followed by a consult with Dr T, and Wednesdays, the day for visiting allied health. As it's too soon into my treatment, I have little to say to Dr T this first visit. She will be more useful in a few weeks' time when the effects of radiation make themselves felt. Tara, the occupational therapist, is different. Radiation can cause lymphoedema in one in four breast cancer patients and it is Tara's job to monitor for any symptoms. Like Jenny, the physio at Tweed Hospital, Tara also has a fancy machine, which soon declares I am a model patient with no apparent symptoms of lymphoedema yet. 'Although,' Tara mentions on examining me, 'you do have some cording.'

Cording, cord-like structures that run from your armpit under the skin on your inner-arm and also known as axillary web syndrome, can occur weeks, months or years after any type of breast surgery. Thought to be caused by inflammation and scarring, they can be painful, although not in my case.

'I can feel it,' I reply. 'But it hasn't really bothered me. I'm trying to do yoga exercises daily, which may be helping.'

Tara agrees that this daily yoga routine is undoubtedly helping and also recommends that I gently massage and stretch the cord.

'It may eventually disappear, or it may just snap one day. You will feel it if it does.'

Like with Dr T, there is not much Kiki, the effervescent allied health nurse can do this soon into my treatment. 'Just make sure you keep applying the Epaderm Cream. Down the track when it gets worse, I'll give you something stronger to use.' Grateful that there will be stronger options later on should I require them, what I don't tell Kiki is, along with the Epaderm Cream, I've also been using some others. Most mainstream health practitioners prefer mainstream treatments, which is why I don't mention it, but I've also done my own research into treating radiation burns. Aloe vera, calendula and chamomile water are frequently mentioned and so I've concocted a potion from these. Applied in tandem with the Epaderm Cream, my chest is so far responding well.

Addendum

Infra-Red Saunas - Unlike regular saunas which use heat to warm the air, infrared saunas heat your body directly. I have purchased (from *Amazon)*, an infrared sauna blanket and found that my body feels not only more relaxed and pliable after using it, but my chest area is less swollen. I also know it is helping me sweat out any toxins.

CHAPTER
20

Finishing Active Treatment

⌇

SHORTLY INTO MY RADIATION TREATMENT, I have my first personal brush with a breast cancer death since my diagnosis. I never met Diane, but we had corresponded a few times via *Messenger* and *Instagram*. A friend of a friend, she had reached out to me earlier on offering advice based on her own breast cancer experience. Also diagnosed with lobular carcinoma, Diane unfortunately had the added blow of her cancer being triple negative. Only 34 with two very young children, Diane fought hard for two years, utilising both conventional and nonconventional treatment methods, but her cancer always appeared to have the upper hand evidenced by her *Instagram* posts. Photos showing her increasingly emaciated frame had saddened me and, after not hearing from her for a period, I wondered if the worst had happened. Today, her page is flooded with messages of farewell and love, so I know she has died. As I said, I never met her personally, but this doesn't make her passing any less tragic, painful or sorrowful to me.

While radiation is incredibly taxing on the body, I can feel myself slowly getting a little stronger. Week by week I can do a little more, although some days I come crashing down and, apart from our morning coffee, spend the rest of the day on the couch. Unlike chemotherapy, which caused mental and physical fatigue along with nausea, radiation leaves me mainly drained with aching legs and groin. My *Women's Cancer Support - GC* group mentions a place just down the coast from us in Kingscliff, Wigs for Wendy. Run by a family who lost their sister to breast cancer, they offer free wigs to cancer patients. One afternoon following radiation, hoping to have a little fun and cheer myself up, I visit this shop and try on various wigs. Despite the amusement of seeing how I could look with short, long, red, black or even purple hair, I depart not having chosen one. I'm comfortable with how my hair is progressing and for the time being, I'll stick with wearing my cap.

Some other afternoons, if I am up to it, are spent following the wide cycle path that traces the Gold Coast coastline on our new scooters. This pathway running from Kingscliff in the south to Southport in the north is perfect for scooter riding and because it's located right alongside the beach, often we will see migrating whales or surf-riding dolphins as we ride. One Sunday morning, we load the scooters into the back of our car and drive to Surfers Paradise. Here, we spend the morning exploring the area before finishing with lunch at the Southport spit. It's the most strenuous thing I have done in months, and it feels great, although, 'It's ridiculous that we can only use our scooters in Queensland,' I whinge to Darryl later that evening.

Electric scooters, we learnt shortly before purchasing them, are forbidden in New South Wales.

'It would be good to utilise the whole cycleway, not just the Queensland part. To be able to ride our scooters at Brunswick Heads. Hopefully, the New South Wales government sees sense, realises that electric scooters can be handy, and eventually removes the ban.'

'It would be good if they were at least treated equally with electric bikes,' Darryl responds. 'They are not subjected to such strict conditions.'

As frequently mentioned by Dr Martin, now that chemotherapy has finished, I'm due for another chest CT scan and brain MRI.

'For the time being, we need to monitor both your chest and brain,' he reminds me in his office one afternoon. 'It will allow us to keep track of any changes. Brain tumours are not really my field, so I'll be referring you to someone whose department it is and sending your scans to them. I'll still be monitoring what's in your chest, though.'

'Who will you be referring me to?'

'Dr Stephenson, a neurosurgeon on the coast.'

'I know her,' I reply, surprised. 'Darryl saw her a few years ago for his back.'

'Yes, she's also a spinal surgeon.'

Still amused that I will be seeing one of Darryl's doctors, a doctor we both hold in great stead, it's a moment or two before I can bring my attention back to Dr Martin.

'I'll write you out a script for letrozole now. It's available from any chemist and you can begin the week after radiation ends,' he is saying.

'Letrozole?' I query.

'Your hormone blocker. You'll need to be on it for eight years.'

Hormone blockers, referred to as hormone therapy, are drugs used to treat hormone positive cancers such as mine. They work by blocking the body's ability to produce hormones, thus depriving breast cancer cells of the fuel (hormones) they use to grow. They are also very effective in reducing cancer spread. Depending on your menopausal status, you could be prescribed a hormone blocker such as tamoxifen (used for both pre- and post-menopausal women), or for post-menopausal women with a higher risk of reoccurrence, a type of hormone blocking drug called an aromatase inhibitor, an example of this being letrozole.

'Are there any side-effects?'

'Everyone's different, but the normal side effects of hormone therapy are like menopausal symptoms. Hot flushes, night sweats, loss of libido, joint and muscle pain, fatigue. Some experience anxiety and mood swings. Because aromatase inhibitors reduce the amount of oestrogen made in the body, this can reduce bone density and put you at risk of osteoporosis and fractures. To reduce this risk, we prescribe denosumab, Prolia. It's an injection you give yourself in the stomach every six months. It's expensive but because it can also give you a very slight advantage in preventing bone metastasis, important. I'll write you out a script for that as well.'

'Does this have any side-effects?'

'The primary side effect is bone and joint pain. In some rare cases, there have been known to be problems with the jaw following tooth extraction. Sometimes users develop a skin rash.'

Leaving Dr Martins' office, I have a lot to think about. I'm already suffering from many of the side-effects he has described, in particular night sweats and fatigue. To hear that my new hormone medication will most likely exacerbate these and learn they will be continuing for the following eight years, along with joint and muscle pain, is disheartening. The further loss of libido doesn't sit well, either. While Darryl and I used to have a very healthy sex life, these days I'm struggling. Something that used to come naturally is now something I am having to work on, fortunately, however, I have avoided the more serious sexual effects that can be caused by chemotherapy such as pelvic pain and vaginal atrophy (the drying, thinning and inflammation of the vaginal walls). I'm also a little worried about the Prolia injections. Not only will they be contributing to the body pain brought about by the aromatase inhibitor, but this drug could also cause my jaw to rot.

'I know I'm going to have to take these drugs,' I cry ruefully to Darryl. 'And I will. As I've said previously, I'm going to do absolutely everything I can to beat this. I just don't want to.'

I'm fortunate to get a combined appointment for my chest CT and brain MRI. It means that immediately following radiation one Wednesday; I make my way to South Coast Radiology, also located at John Flynn Hospital. I've had an interesting morning. While the radiation treatment procedure has become second nature, lie on the table, open my gown, be pushed into place, deep breath, leave— every radiation session finds a different crew manning the machines, some more diligent than others. This morning's team were the most conscientious yet, pushing and prodding until I was positioned exactly right, leaving the room to check from their safe observation point, then returning to move me a fraction more. I also had something to show Kiki, the allied health care nurse.

'My chest hasn't blistered, but it is looking red and raw and is painful,' I mention, taking off my top.

'Where are you up to? Session 19,' she murmurs, consulting my notes. 'You're exactly where I would expect you to be. It starts to get a bit more inflamed about now. The worse will occur a week to 10 days following your last session. I'll give you this to try. It's cortisone-based, so it's much more effective in controlling the burn.'

Apart from some difficulty inserting the cannula, my scans are straight-forward. Perhaps because of a build-up of scar tissue, but it takes three attempts to insert the needle into the vein of my right arm. I've been told to only use my right-arm, the arm where lymph nodes were not removed, when having needles or my blood pressure taken, as using my left arm could cause lymphoedema. Although I later find out this information has been proven incorrect, I and a lot of other breast cancer patients I know, still follow this practice.

I'm at my YWCA Encore class when Doc Martin phones with the results. I can't take the call as I am fully engrossed in this week's presentation. Contrary to what Kim, our instructor, had told us earlier, the Dragon Boat ladies did not appear during week two, rather they are here today, giving this week's session. Apart from Kim, I'm the only one who has managed to make it to this week's class, and I don't want to let the Dragon Boat ladies down by taking a phone call.

Dragon Boat racing came to be linked to breast cancer I learn, back in 1995 when Dr Don McKenzie, seeking to debunk the myth that breast cancer survivors should avoid strenuous activities to prevent lymphoedema, settled on Dragon Boat racing to make his point. Putting together a team of women who had undergone breast cancer, their training and subsequent competing in events produced interesting results. There were no cases of lymphoedema, and every lady could show a marked improvement in her mental and physical health. Dragon Boat racing and breast cancer have become synonymous ever since.

'Your scans all look fine,' Doc Martin reassures me a short time after class has finished. 'No change since last time. I've also got some other news. I've just received an email about a new drug, abemaciclib or Verzenio. It belongs to a group of drugs that blocks kinase, the protein that helps cells grow and divide. Block kinase and you can stop cancer cells growing and dividing. They have been running trials overseas and have seen some excellent results. Now they have opened the program to just 300 Australian breast cancer patients who meet certain criteria. These patients must be about to start or have just begun hormone therapy, must have at least four involved axillary lymph nodes or if they have less than three lymph nodes involved, then they must be stage 3 or have a tumour of at least 5 cm.'

'I meet all of those requirements,' I interrupt.

'Normally, this drug would cost in the tens of thousands of dollars. This program is offering it to 300 Australians for free. There are side-effects, such as fatigue, but the main one seems to be diarrhoea.'

'That's fine,' I interrupt again. 'Just get me on it.'

Wednesday, 21 September, my last day of radiation. Memorable because it's Darryl's father's birthday. I am meant to be finishing tomorrow, but that's a public holiday and Genesis Care does not open on public holidays. Determined to finish as soon as possible, I have organised to have two radiation sessions today rather than wait until Friday. If I leave a gap of at least six hours between the two appointments, according to Dr T, it should be fine.

It's been a week of contrasts. I'm happily celebrating the end of active treatment. It will be tablets from here on in, but mum's in hospital trying to work out what heart mediations work best for her. She has declined rapidly over the past month, and we are really hoping this hospital visit will provide some benefit. That she will find the medication that she needs. After nearly five months, I've finally discarded my cap. My hair has grown enough that I'm comfortable to show it to the universe, and shortly both Darryl and I will throw away our masks. We can finally join the real world, meet up with family, go places. But I'm shattered, my chest is fire-engine red, raw, oozy and itchy, expected to get worse before it gets better, and my hot flashes are going mad. I'm having huge surges of heat day and night and I haven't even started the hormone blockers yet. Doc Martin has advised that I have been accepted into the abemaciclib program, which I am ecstatic about, but the diarrhoea stories I have been reading in a dedicated Verzenio *Facebook* support group are horrendous. Tales of ladies having to carry a potty in their car or having to wear adult diapers have me really concerned, although, fortunately, there are more pleasant stories; some patients have suffered only a few side-effects. I'm determined to be one of these.

Walking into Northern Rivers, the crew know it's my last session, the end of 25 rounds of radiation preceded by five months of chemotherapy, two mastectomy operations, an infection, and congratulate me accordingly.

'Come on, let's get this over and done with.' Then later. 'Congratulations. Well done. Now get out of here.'

Kiki is required to see me before I leave the building, and Dr T checks in as well. Both warn me that the following 10 days will be the worst.

'I'm giving you this extra cream and some padding plus some saline,' Kiki tells me.

'Drench the padding with the saline and place it over your burn. Leave for 10 minutes, then apply the cream. It will help.'

Dr T just nods in satisfaction and says she will see me in a week's time.

As expected, over the following week, the burn on my chest and under my arm progressively gets worse. Chaffed, weepy, swollen, and painful, I'm fortunate that I don't lose too many layers of skin, nor the skin split too deeply. I've seen photos where radiation has caused profound cracking—a serious infection concern. I'm putting my avoidance of this more severe outcome down to Kiki's fantastic cream, the saline soaked padding and my own home-made concoction. I visit Dr T twice more over this period before, on 30 September, she wishes me well and tells me she hopes she never sees me again.

Addendum

Tumour marker tests - Following treatment some breast cancer warriors like to keep an eye on the results of certain cancer marker tests – cancer antigen 15-3, cancer antigen 27.29 and carcinoembryonic (CEA). Mainstream practitioners advocate that these tests are not useful in detecting cancer recurrence or in lengthening life. I get them for my own peace of mind.

CHAPTER
21

Hormone Therapy

———

IT'S OCTOBER NOW, 10 MONTHS since diagnosis, 10 months since Dr Taylor uttered those heart stopping words, 'it's breast cancer', that so changed my life. Active treatment—chemotherapy and radiation has finished, but the battle isn't over. Fittingly, I heard a great analogy recently that sums up a breast cancer journey—my journey. It likened breast cancer to a diseased tree. Following diagnosis, first, comes the chainsaw, the mastectomy, to cut down the tree and remove the rot. Then comes the bulldozer or chemotherapy to clear up the bigger mess that's been left behind, the branches, twigs and leaves—the cancer cells. But the bulldozer and chemo can't get rid of the tiny particles still left in the soil or in your body. That's where the rake, the radiation, comes in. To target those minute cells still floating around. Finally, there's the weed killers like letrozole, tamoxifen, Faslodex and abemaciclib. These, hopefully, stop a new tree, a new cancer from growing.

I've faced the chainsaw, the bulldozer, the rake. Now it's time for the weed killers. In my case, these will be letrozole, which I will be on for the next eight years, and abemaciclib, also known as Verzenio, for the next two.

I start on the letrozole first. It requires a prescription and I can only get a fresh packet every 28 days, no bulk buying allowed. Prior to my visit to a chemist, I do a little online research and following the advice of fellow users, I've made sure to procure the Sandoz brand because, 'it has way fewer side-effects,' apparently. I've yet to try any other brand so I'm not sure if this advice is correct or not.

Seven days after finishing radiation, I take my first letrozole tablet and seven days after that, my first abemaciclib (interestingly, a two-month's supply of abemaciclib just turns up in the mail one day and will continue to do so for another 22 months). This was a few weeks ago and since then, I've been feeling pretty awful. Any body aches and pains I had prior, have increased tenfold and I'm putting this down to the estrogen leaching (estrogen protects joints and reduces inflammation), letrozole. While it's a 24-hour problem, the worst occurs at night with joint aches very reminiscent of childhood growing pains, waking me multiple times.

I'm blaming some other issues, namely nausea and lethargy, on the abemaciclib. Feeling queasy immediately after taking my first dose, it was easy to pinpoint this as the culprit. While it's been tolerable in the evening, when I can take a tablet just before bed and can thus sleep through its stomach churning effects, the morning pill is different. Every morning since I began, I have felt sick, nearly as bad as when I was going through chemotherapy. Eating breakfast is once again difficult and although, thank goodness, I've only had mild diarrhoea; I have noticed a huge escalation in fatigue, common with my current dosage, apparently. Any physical gains made over the past few months have been lost, as I've also been finding it really difficult to summon the strength to go on my daily walks. When I do, I find them much harder, often returning home breathless and exhausted. Doc Martin has said if the effects get too bad, I can reduce to a lower dosage, but I will try hard to avoid doing so. As I have said many times before, I am going to do absolutely everything I can to fight this breast cancer. I read somewhere that the best remedy for both joint pain and fatigue is exercise. I'll obviously just have to try harder. Fight the weariness. Push through my yoga stretches.

As predicted by Kiki and Dr T, my radiation burn, a few weeks post treatment, is finally beginning to abate, now a fierce pink, it looks much better than the weeping crimson it was. It's fortunate timing because spring is here, the weather is warming, and it's much nicer to be wearing looser, cooler, more comfortable clothing as we slowly reintegrate into the wider world. It was hard eliminating the safety blanket that our masks became, but they have gone. A fact noticed by Cara when I turn up for yet another blood test.

'So that's what you look like underneath your cap and mask,' she laughs.

'It definitely feels strange not wearing something on my face,' I reply. 'Although I will probably never get rid of my hand sanitiser,' said as I pull it from my pocket.

'I didn't think I would see you again so soon, seeing as you've finished treatment.'

'I've just started on letrozole, and a new drug called abemaciclib. Fortnightly, then monthly, then tri-monthly blood tests are a requirement of abemaciclib for the first year. So, you will see me for a while yet.'

Which she does as over the following month, I slowly rebuild a life post active breast cancer treatment, post Covid. Because of the body aches and fatigue, it's challenging, but I start with the things I have missed the most. Things so enjoyable that how I feel is pushed aside. Something like a three-day visit to my daughter in Brisbane. Visiting Paige and it feels incredible after an almost three-year hiatus, to be once again catching public transport, mingling in large malls, shopping. We spend one day ogling elephants at Australia Zoo on the Sunshine Coast, another navigating various Brisbane suburbs on hired electric scooters. My final morning is spent hunting for a vacuum cleaner for our little Coolangatta unit. Unfortunately, my foray back into life doesn't come without a cost, though. Journeying home by train, I note that my lower back feels sore, an ache that progressively worsens over the following week until I am forced to visit a chiropractor.

'Muscle weakness is a common side-effect of chemotherapy and radiation,' I learn. 'Your body has been exposed to a lot over the past six months. It's not surprising that you have some soft-tissue pain. Radiation and chemotherapy can affect soft-tissue, muscles, ligaments and skin.'

My suppleness and endurance, I realise, are just other things cancer has robbed me of.

A fact corroborated when, a few weeks later, I reintroduce another missed activity, my lawn bowls. Whereas once spending all day bowling came easily, now I struggle to finish one game. It doesn't stop me, however, thoroughly enjoying myself, happy to be back amongst great friends.

November passes and December arrives, a year since that initial revealing mammogram and ultrasound. This year something different marks December, Covid. It's laughable, really. After being so diligent for so many months with our mask wearing, hand sanitising and isolating, I end up catching it at my end-of-year Women Bowlers' Christmas party, of all places. I catch it from Pauline, that fellow cancer survivor who

I mentioned earlier. Because she gets such a bad dose and spends the week following the party in bed, she doesn't inform anyone that she is sick. When I start to display symptoms, I don't consider it could be Covid but take a test, anyway. It comes back negative. The following day I feel worse, so take another test. Again, it comes back negative. That night, feeling pretty miserable, I present at Byron Bay Hospital where a more sensitive PCR test is administered prior to me being sent home. The following morning, the result appears via text on my phone, positive. Fortunately, I am able to access antiviral meds and, by day five, feel almost completely well again. While I am relieved to finally have Covid over and done with, it did arrive at an unfortunate time. An appointment with Dr Stephenson, the neurosurgeon who will be monitoring my brain tumour, has had to be postponed until February, as has an appointment with Dr Binjemain. Dr Binjemain is the integrative doctor familiar with the Jane McLelland protocol and after a six-month wait, finally has a spot for me. Fortunately, I am able to reschedule this appointment for early in the new year.

Addendum

Environmental Toxins – It's taken a diagnosis of breast cancer to awaken me to the amount of chemicals I have been subjecting myself to. Dosing myself daily with perfume, makeup, shampoo, cleansers, toners and body lotions, I'm drowning in harmful toxins. Add the ones I eat, drink and breathe, it's no wonder my body rebelled. Give some thought to the chemicals you're exposing yourself to.

CHAPTER
22

Re-Embracing Life

—⁓—

12 JANUARY 2023, MY ONE-YEAR cancerversary. I'm back at John Flynn Hospital, but this time, it's to accompany my mother as she meets with her heart specialist. Despite a worsening of her COPD, she's still hanging in there. She's as frail as a baby bird and she sounds like she's breathing through a blocked straw, but she's a Kiwi and as tough as they come. All we learn at this appointment is that there is nothing more they can do for her and to appreciate the time she has left. Always one to enjoy having a good time; an impromptu party, no doubt, is what she has in mind.

My appointment with Dr Binjemain has finally arrived and coincidentally, it's on the same day that local news channels are spruiking the news that they have allocated two McGrath Breast Care nurses to the Gold Coast region. While on the face of it, the news sounds great, what they aren't telling us and what I have learnt via my *Women's Cancer*

Support - GC group is that these two nurses are being plucked from a pool of existing breast care nurses. They are actually current breast care nurses being relabelled as McGrath nurses. Actual breast care nurse numbers will stay exactly the same. It's very frustrating.

My visit to Dr Binjemain, however, is the complete opposite. His office is located near the Robina Town Centre shopping precinct, and after a quick visit there, both Darryl and I attend the two-hour appointment. While the first 60 minutes are taken up with discussing the various causes of cancer, because of his privacy policy, I cannot go into his theories here. They are nonetheless, 100% believable and heavily based on the toxicities, both environmental and behavioural, we expose ourselves to. We spend the second hour working on how I can further support my own fight against cancer.

'Because you are nearly six-months post chemotherapy treatment, I don't advocate Jane's drugs for you,' he tells me. 'Metformin, doxycycline, mebendazole, dipyridamole. These are best taken immediately after treatment or if you were stage 4. Instead, I would look at increasing your white blood cell count, which is being negatively affected by the medications you are currently taking, letrozole and abemaciclib. This will reduce any infection risk and generally make you feel a bit better. Thymosin alpha could help. You said abemaciclib causes fatigue. There are alternative remedies you could try, like methylene blue and PQQ.'

'And the current supplements I am taking,' handing him my long list. 'Are they ok?'

'Just swop the K2 and D3 around. K2 is better taken in the morning, while D3 should be taken later in the day.'

It's an extensive and detailed appointment and too much is discussed to disclose everything here, but I leave his office with a much greater awareness of my environment and behaviours. I need to be even more vigilant about the toothpaste I use, the moisturisers I rub into my body, the detergents I buy, the food I eat, the water I drink.

'Some methods of eliminating toxins from our body,' Dr Binjemain finishes with, 'are coffee enemas, infrared saunas or undertaking a niacin detox.' A niacin detox, I learn, is a procedure whereby I would take a dose of niacin, exercise, then have a sauna. As our Coolangatta property has a sauna, it's something Darryl and I both vow to do. The coffee enemas, I'll build up to.

February arrives, as does my appointment with Dr Ellison, my neurosurgeon. Prior to my visit, she has sent me to an optician for testing and today we discuss the results.

'The tumour is affecting the vision in your left eye; it's affected the sight in this lower quadrant. All we can do for the time being is keep an eye on it with regular brain scans and optician appointments to monitor any further loss of sight. Your options, should it enlarge further, are radiation or surgery.'

It's a blow hearing this news, but I am not surprised. I've actually noticed the deterioration in my sight. It's become more difficult to see the jack when I bowl, and the computer screen often looks blurry as I type. What this news does though, is it reminds me and reinforces what I said to Darryl during that difficult conversation some months ago. Having cancer, not knowing if I am going to be alive in four, five or ten years' time, not knowing if something else like deteriorating eyesight, is going to come along, means, I need to live my life now.

As so often happens when you decide on something, something else occurs that aids your decision. One morning, shortly after my appointment with Dr Stephenson, an email arrives advertising a cheap repositioning cruise on Richard Branson's new and aptly named ship, the Resilient Lady. Departing Sydney in late March 2024, it will relocate to Athens via South-East Asia, India and the Suez Canal. As it also contains a visit to Egypt, a country I have always wanted to visit, within a fortnight, we have not only booked this cruise, but put in motion, steps to visit both Turkey and Israel. All going to plan, May and June 2024 should see me really living my life by crossing both Istanbul and Jerusalem off my ever-evolving Bucket List. While the itinerary is a little tamer than our previous travels, it feels incredible booking this new journey, like I'm really committing to the future and putting this tiring cancer adventure behind me. As do some other long held goals, achievements designed more for self-fulfilment and growth, rather than travel, which I'm ready to implement.

The first is to sign up to the University of the 3rd Age, a university I first heard about from my Aunt Cherry and a university, once I turned 50, that I wanted to attend. Coolangatta, I discover, has one of these campuses and an online search of its classes, reveal it's of a high calibre. It's easy enough to enrol and within a few weeks, one undertaking on my list has been fulfilled when I find myself sitting with a host of other like-minded individuals enjoying both history and art history lessons.

The second goal I start aiming for is to become a Gold Coast Airport Ambassador. It's a volunteer role and involves undergoing a training program that would see me, one shift a week, assisting passengers at the busy airport. Loving travel as I do, I think I would enjoy the tension of a high security airport, being thrust amongst other travellers, helping them when need be. I have been advised that another training intake is happening shortly and so I put my name down for that.

The third item on my list that needs to begin is a new book. The book that's been mulling around in my head for the past 12 months. This book. I've learnt a lot on this breast cancer adventure and I need to pass it on. Not only to other breast cancer survivors, but to the public at large. I'm sure there are many out there who have not the slightest inkling of what a diagnosis of breast cancer actually entails. I've been taking notes, worked out the first part, my adventure, the story you have just read. Now, I'm going to spend the next few autumn months, March, April and May, working on part two, stories from other fighters, other survivors. I'm going to meet with them and over a coffee or two, listen and learn. I feel that if anyone can teach us anything about surviving and living with breast cancer, then it's these amazing ladies fighting on the front line.

Addendum

Look after yourself - Ask about Medicare Enhanced Primary Care plans. Book into a Look Good Feel Better workshop. Investigate whether the YWCA Encore program is happening near you. Treat yourself to a good coffee (if you're a coffee drinker). Think about separate bed coverings. Have a lymphatic drainage massage. Eat healthily. Exercise.

PART TWO

Their Stories

CHAPTER
23

Tracey-Triple Negative Stage 3

<hr>

TRACEY, DIAGNOSED WITH STAGE 3 triple negative cancer in February 2020, is my experimental subject, the first person I meet with to get their story. It's mid-morning on what appears to be pension day, as the café we have chosen is thronged with elderly pensioners happily chatting away. She's had to put the time of our meeting back, because, that morning, she's accompanied her husband to his own follow up oncologist appointment. But I'll get to that later. Despite the timing hiccup and the noise, I soon find myself engrossed in Tracey's tale.

One morning Tracey, a 56-year-old former general manager of an aged care home, now because of lifestyle choices, an assistant manager at the same venue, woke and, while having her morning shower, felt a noticeable lump under her arm.

'I'm not sure how long it had been there, but that morning I felt a definite lump. Something didn't feel right.'

Managing to get a mammogram and an ultrasound appointment within two days, as I will increasingly discover, the mammogram showed nothing, but the ultrasound warranted a follow up biopsy.

'I was lucky. The technician performing my ultrasound that day was the head guy. He could also perform my biopsy, which he did that same afternoon.'

'So, you got all your tests done within two days of feeling a lump?'

'Yes.'

Tracey's biopsy revealed it was breast cancer, although she wasn't aware what type until she met with her breast and endocrine specialist a few weeks later and was told she had triple negative breast cancer, stage 3. She also learnt that it had spread to her lymph nodes and because her tumour was so large, her doctor was advocating chemotherapy first, then surgery, followed by radiation and maybe, due to it being triple negative, a second round of oral chemotherapy.

'And this is what you did?'

'Yes. At first there were some feelings of denial, but then I realised that this was what it is. This was happening. I had to do what I had to do. I had to get rid of it.'

'Where did you do your chemotherapy and do you remember what regime you were on?'

'At John Flynn Hospital.' Tracey replies. 'I met with my oncologist and he straight out told me he wasn't going to lie. That triple negative was one of the worst to get and to not Google anything. That the statistics were bad. I started treatment right at the beginning of Covid. My husband and daughter could accompany me the first few times, but that was eventually stopped because of Covid's restrictions. I had to go on my own from then onwards. I had the four Red Devils followed by the paclitaxel.'

'How did you find chemo?'

Tracey's answer to this question utterly surprises me and gives me my first inkling into just how tough, how strong a fighter she is.

'Not that bad. I kept working while I underwent treatment.'

As I sit listening, slightly incredulous, after all I've just gone through this same chemo regime albeit after surgery, Tracey goes on to explain how she managed to continue working at a busy aged care centre whilst undergoing treatment for cancer. The system she adopted, she tells me, was to have her Red Devil (doxorubicin) on a Thursday morning, go home and sleep all afternoon in a darkened room. 'I would then spend all day Friday in bed and some of Saturday. Sundays, I was starting to feel a bit better and by Monday, I was ready to return to work.' As her doxorubicin was administered fortnightly, Tracey found this arrangement worked well for her.

'The Taxol was different though,' she muses. 'Because it was weekly, I changed my treatment to Wednesday mornings. I would have my chemo, then go home and sleep all afternoon, then return to work on Thursday. Everyone there knew they were not allowed to contact me on Wednesdays. Although as time went by, I started taking some work into chemo and would answer emails and sometimes make phone calls from my chair. I found that working kept my mind off things. It made me feel useful, and it helped me get through it.'

'I can understand that work would have distracted you and helped you get through chemo, but I don't know how you found the energy to do it. Work is the last thing I could have done. How about your surgery?' I quiz. 'Did you have a mastectomy? Lumpectomy?'

'I had a single mastectomy. Although my jaw dropped when my doctor gave me my surgery date. It was 22 July 2020. Seven years to the day that I had my stroke.'

'You've had a stroke?'

'Yes.'

Seven years ago, Tracey was camping with her family when she woke one morning feeling tingly down one side.

'Like there was a line down the middle of me with pins and needles on this one side.'

Walking around her campsite, preparing breakfast, Tracey found herself tripping over guy-ropes and generally feeling that something wasn't right.

'I had my daughter take me to hospital. When I told them my symptoms, they had me in a wheelchair and into a bed straight away.'

Tracey spent 10 days in hospital and her treatment was aspirin.

'The worst bit was that they couldn't tell me what had caused it. I did every test on earth, but they couldn't give me a reason. They did mutter something about the pill, but they couldn't be sure.'

'How long did the pins and needles last?' I ask. 'Were they temporary?'

'No. They lasted ages, and it was years before my underarm on one side felt normal again. Probably what helped me was my dancing. I do tap, jazz and cabaret dancing. So does my daughter. We had a dance concert coming up. It was probably about six weeks after I had my stroke and I said that I was still going to do the concert. And I did. It nearly killed me, but I did it. I was determined to. The doctors mentioned it was probably my brain dealing with the jazz co-ordination that helped it recover so quickly and the exercise helped with my body.'

'So, you had your surgery,' I prompt, returning to my questions.

'Yes. I had a single mastectomy. I had this just when my husband got diagnosed with prostate then kidney cancer. He needed two operations, so we ended up having to juggle three surgeries and then my radiation.'

Lending weight to my assertion that this is one incredibly strong, decisive lady, Tracey proceeds to tell me calmly that while undergoing perhaps the biggest fight of her life, she also had to support her husband through not one, but two cancer diagnoses.

'They discovered his prostate cancer first, and it was during these tests that they discovered the kidney cancer. He had his prostrate removed, then a second operation. With so many operations, I decided against reconstruction. The tummy tuck would have been good, but I just didn't want to face hospital again.'

'How is your husband now?'

'He just needs two new knees now.'

'And your radiation. How did that go?'

'It was fine. I had it at John Flynn Hospital. Sandra from the *Gold Coast Cancer support* group was good here. She advised me to question the amount they were going to charge me. I ended up getting it for nothing. The worst thing about radiation was the New South Wales and Queensland border closure because of Covid.'

Tracey's radiation timeframe, it turns out, occurred right when the Queensland government closed its border to New South Wales. It meant Tracey was required to print out special medical passes and allow herself plenty of additional time in order to get from her home in New South Wales, to John Flynn Hospital in Queensland. It made a difficult time even harder.

'Although, in hindsight, it probably wasn't the worse time to be going through treatment for breast cancer. While I couldn't go anywhere because of my treatment, no one else was going anywhere either because of Covid. At least I wasn't missing out on things.'

'Are you still working full time?'

'No. With my husband requiring his surgeries, and mine, I ended up taking about 15 months off. I had to. I was exhausted. I did return to work four days a week as a revolving general manager, but that position was later made full-time, something I didn't want to do. Luckily, they then created an assistant manager's position, which I could do four days a week and which I am still doing now. These days I use Fridays, the day I don't work, to attend appointments such as lymphoedema physiotherapy, my oncology follow-ups and my husband's follow-up appointments, which is where I was earlier.'

Because Tracey's cancer is triple negative, following radiation treatment, she is not offered a hormone blocker such as letrozole that those with hormone positive cancers are.

'My oncologist told me I was one of the lucky ones because I wouldn't have to suffer any of the side effects those drugs can cause.'

We both have a bit of a laugh over this. Both understanding the irony of calling someone battling triple negative cancer, lucky.

'I did have to go through another round of chemotherapy following radiation, although this time I took tablets. Funny enough, I found the side-effects from this chemo even worse than when it was administered via my port, which I still have, by the way. This second lot of chemo caused my feet to blister so badly that I could only wear really soft thongs.'

'It's been just over three years now since your diagnosis. Have you learnt anything from your journey? Have you made any lifestyle changes?'

'We had bought a caravan before I was diagnosed. Now we are determined to use it. To travel. There are a few things we need to organise first. Sell our business—we have a pool business. My husband needs to get his knees operated on, then we can reassess. But we will definitely travel more.'

'I can certainly relate to that. So, I've just a couple more questions. Did you learn anything that you could offer someone newly diagnosed?'

'Paint your nails a dark colour before chemo. I made sure I did this. I painted them a really dark purple and my fingernails stayed strong and healthy. But I forgot to look after my toes, and I lost all my toenails. What I would also tell someone newly diagnosed is to take one step at a time. You're going to be overwhelmed with information and procedures. Just concentrate on the first step when that's done, then think about the next one. I've also learnt to stay positive. Scream and cry when or if you need to, but stay positive.'

'You sound like someone who has things happen to them, but you just deal with it?'

'That's true. That's why I need to stay positive. It's who I am. Although I hated losing my hair. I think I found that the hardest part of all this. I found it really difficult to stay positive when I lost it. I wore scarves and hats, but my hair was part of me. My identity.'

'So, last question. That was advice for someone newly diagnosed with cancer. Is there anything you can offer, any advice to give, to those without cancer?'

'That's a hard one,' Tracey replies. 'But I could suggest that they don't assume to know what we are going through, what it's like to have cancer. I've had this happen. I've also had people comparing me to someone else with cancer. Everyone's cancer is different. Everyone reacts to it differently. So don't assume that because this happened to so and so, that it's the same with me. Also, I've had people talk about how they know someone who died from cancer. Don't go there. I don't want to hear this. And I could also tell them that cancer can happen to anyone. It doesn't discriminate.'

Wrapping up the interview, Tracey tells me a brief story, her words perhaps the most poignant, certainly the most insightful, so far.

'I have a 28-year-old daughter who was in a stable relationship for seven years. I would often get asked, 'so when are the grandkids due?' which would really annoy me. Grandkids were something none of us thought about. They were part of a far-off future. It's different now. I just want to still be here to see my daughter married. I can't wait for grandkids now.'

For my first interview, I've found it incredibly interesting and informative. I'm still surprised that Tracey managed to keep working whilst undergoing treatment (she will eventuate to be one of only two people I meet who do so) and I've enjoyed sitting one on one just chatting about our respective breast cancer journeys. Introducing other ladies' stories for comparison with my own, I feel, is going to be educational and the success of this first interview means I am looking forward to getting more.

Addendum

Nails - Chemotherapy attacks fast growing cells. As your nail cells fall into this category, chemo can have an adverse effect on them. They can cause them to weaken, split and even fall off. Patients are often advised to paint their nails with a protective, strengthening polish before commencing treatment. While my nails didn't fall off, they did become weak and brittle. Something still occurring 15 months after chemo due to the abemaciclib (which also attacks fast growing cells) I am currently taking.

CHAPTER
24

Karen-HER2 Stage 4

KAREN IS A CALM, THOUGHTFUL 66-year-old who joined the cancer roller coaster in September 2022. Diagnosed stage 4 (metastasised) HER2 positive, I catch up with Karen one Saturday morning. I'm running late for our meeting, but true to her gracious nature, Karen asks me not to apologise. 'What does being a little late matter? In the scheme of things, being late is so unimportant. I was fine waiting.'

I am grateful for Karen's understanding, and even more so when I hear her story.

Back in December 2021, Karen lost her 90-year-old mum and was sorting through her things, cleaning out her house, when she felt a 'tremendous pain in her back. I was in agony. Could hardly walk. Lying down was impossible, and I ended up sleeping in mum's recliner.'

Putting it down to a bad back strain, Karen endured the discomfort for months.

'I was busy with mum's house. We had some issues with the will. My older brother wanted to contest it, so I was really stressed. I just kept putting off going to a doctor.'

Eventually, early September 2022, some 10 months later, when Karen also noticed pain occurring across her chest region, she made an appointment to see a GP.

'He organised for me to have an x-ray. I got the results of the x-ray by email. It said that the radiologist had spotted something in my lymph nodes and that I needed more tests.'

More tests eventuated to be a chest CT and a breast biopsy.

'When I went for the breast biopsy, they were meant to be biopsying both sides, but when they took the first sample and tested it, I could hear the nurse talking. She was saying, "Oh, look how quickly that has turned. It's turned really milky." I knew straight away that something was wrong. That this was bad.'

Despite her having heard the nurse utter these words and the immediate cancellation of her second biopsy, Karen was sent home, where a week later, on 29 September, she was advised to present for an appointment with an oncologist at her local hospital.

'There were two doctors. I took a friend with me, and they sat me down. They started talking to me as if I was a child. They didn't come out and really say anything; they just kept pussy footing around. Eventually I said to just tell me, and this is when I learnt I had stage 4 cancer. I wanted more information, but all they could give me was a plan of what was to happen next.'

Prior to her diagnosis, Karen had been thinking of travel, 'maybe do an Asian river cruise', but this was all put aside when her 'plan' evolved into blood tests, a PET scan, and a breast MRI.

'The MRI was a nightmare. I was at my local hospital, but I couldn't fit into their machine. I'm a big woman, but I'm not that big. They tried three times, and, in the end, they had to take me by ambulance to another centre. Then on my way back from this scan, I get a phone call from Genesis at John Flynn asking me to come in for my radiation simulation. I knew nothing about this. Had no idea what they were talking about. I hadn't been told I needed radiation.'

From what I am gathering, Karen's initial journey was not a straight-forward one. Definitely lacking in the provision of answers and information. A little more convoluted and confusing than some. One week after finding out she had stage 4 breast cancer, Karen found herself undertaking radiation.

'I was told I only had to do five sessions of radiation and that I was lucky as I would get none of the radiation burns others get.'

'Why only one week of radiation?' I query.

'I think it's because they then got the results of my MRI and PET scans. I had to return to my hospital, and the doctors told me they had found five spots of cancer in my spine and one spot near the back of my head. There were no spots in the breasts, but the pathology from the biopsy said that the spots were metastasised breast cancer. They didn't know where the primary was and they told me because it had spread, I would not need any operations and they also told me I had probably two to four, maybe five years to live.'

'They told you that?'

'Yes. Which is strange really because when my dad died, even though he had cancer right through him, the doctors wouldn't give him a timeframe.'

'Did you need chemotherapy?'

'Yes. So, on 25 October, I had my port inserted in the morning, then that afternoon I had my first chemo. Five days later, on 30 October, I got a blood clot in my arm. I knew it was a blood clot because I got one once before after I had my gall bladder removed. I went to the hospital around 11 pm but didn't get to see a doctor until 4 am. I just sat there all night.'

'I've heard about patients who had their ports inserted in the morning, then had chemo that same day. It wouldn't have been very nice. What happened after you saw a doctor?'

'They gave me two shots of warfarin, then sent me home. I'm still on blood thinners.'

'And chemo. Do you know what regime you were on and for how long?'

'I don't know what drugs they gave me, but I only did chemo for a few weeks, then they stopped it as they didn't think it would work for me.'

'Really. What did you think of that?'

'I think they use chemo, especially in my case, a stage 4, as just a "go to" drug. Something to do just so they are doing something. I am on chemotherapy tablets now though and will be on them forever. I've written them down.'

'Pertuzumab and trastuzumab,' I read aloud.

'Yes. They must be doing something because my most recent PET scan showed the spine spots shrinking. I am also on denosumab. Every four weeks I go back to the hospital and get an injection.'

'Denosumab. That's Prolia, I think. I'm on that as well, but fortunately, I only need it every six months. You've certainly got an incredible story and you've definitely had it tough.

Is there anything you think you have learnt from all this?'

'Definitely. That the little things aren't big things anymore. So what if the house is a little dirty? So what if my son doesn't pick up all his stuff? These little things are not worth stressing over anymore. My friend said he would provide dinner last night. He brought home some pies, and the tops burnt slightly in the oven as he was reheating them. He got really upset and kept apologising. But who cares about a burnt pie?'

'Being stage 4, do others treat you any differently now?'

'Yes. Although this is probably one of the good things. I used to feel like a glorified babysitter. But now my kids are much more appreciative. My sons actually phone and check in on me now and my daughter has been a real help.'

'How about life changes? Do you do anything differently?'

'It's only been seven months and I am still getting myself organised. I've been living with friends while I have been going through this while I get my own home sorted. But I am making time to catch up with friends. To stop and have a coffee. I wear brighter clothing now. I used to only wear black but now I will wear a really colourful top. I've bought colourful joggers. This top is new. Later, I'll start visiting more friends and family.'

'Part of the reason I am writing this book is to provide information to both those newly diagnosed and to those who don't have a clue what we are going through. Is there anything you wish you had been aware of or is there something that would have helped you earlier on in your diagnosis?'

'You get told so much at the beginning and it is all so confusing. I would tell anyone newly diagnosed to bring a friend with them to their consults or at least record everything that is being said. There is too much information overload, and you can just black it all out. I also really wish that someone would put a bag of information together and give it to you when you first get diagnosed. It could have information on scans, what to expect. I don't know. It just would have been so helpful to have more information to read at home.'

It's been a thought-provoking conversation with a fascinatingly courageous warrior. Despite a stage 4 diagnosis with a life expectancy of two to four/five years, Karen is happy and, in her own words, 'lucky.' 'I have my own house, some money in the bank, great friends, supportive family. It's the younger, newly diagnosed ones I feel for. The girls with young children. Compared to them, I'm very lucky.'

Addendum

Magnetic resonance imaging or MRI Scans – Use a strong magnetic field and radio waves to take pictures inside your body. Specifically useful in capturing soft tissue images that don't show up on x-ray, for example, pictures of your muscles and organs. When having a breast MRI – you will lay face down on a table. Taking about 25-30 minutes, the worse bit is the noise the machine makes.

CHAPTER
25

Kelly-Invasive Ductal ER and HER2 Positive

KELLY, A GORGEOUS BUBBLY 44-YEAR-OLD primary school teacher and mother to two young teenage boys, could easily be one of those young mothers Karen has referenced. Diagnosed in February 2023, not all that long ago, with invasive ductal carcinoma, Kelly is undertaking neo-adjuvant therapy, (chemotherapy before surgery) thus is not yet sure of her cancer's stage nor grade. These she expects to get once she has had her mastectomy, and the pathology returned. What her earlier biopsies have revealed is that her cancer is both ER and HER2 positive, PR negative.

'I have three cancerous tumours in my left breast. Two are ER positive, HER2 negative, but the third is HER2 positive,' Kelly tells me. 'Because of my age and the HER2 diagnosis, my treatment will be four to six sessions of chemotherapy, each three weeks apart, then a mastectomy, then probably eleven more rounds of chemo, depends on how I handle it. I was going to just have a lumpectomy but when the third tumour came back HER2 positive, it changed to a mastectomy. I am unsure whether or not I will be having radiation.'

'Then maybe hormone therapy?' I question.

'Yes, then hormone therapy.'

It's a brilliant autumn morning when I meet up with Kelly to hear her story. She has not long had to shave off her hair, and she looks lovely as we sit, chatting over our respective coffee and hot chocolate, her head artfully draped in a chic scarf. As she tells me her tale, parts of it resonate. It's not too dissimilar to mine.

Around 15 years ago, Kelly noticed a few tiny lumps in her left breast. Diagnosed as fibroadenomas, solid, smooth benign lumps commonly found in women in their 20s and 30s, Kelly was advised to keep a close eye on them and to have regular mammograms and ultrasounds, which she did.

'It sounds funny now, but I kind of always thought that I would get breast cancer, so I was always very vigilant, always checking them. When I turned 40, about 10 years after they first appeared, I noticed them getting larger. I could feel them more. In January this year, I visited my doctor who, after also feeling them, sent me for another ultrasound and mammogram. I'm not sure if the three tumours they found with these latest tests were the original three cysts. I would have to check my earlier imaging, but they all came back positive for breast cancer. It was a real blow. This was meant to be my year. My boys and I had just moved into my new partner's house. I had just taken on a new teaching contract, due to begin next term, which dealt with special needs children, something I had wanted to do for years, then I got diagnosed.'

As Kelly mentioned, because of her young age and the HER2 positive component of her diagnosis, it was recommended she undertake chemotherapy first, then surgery.

'Although I did have some lymph nodes removed early on, a lymph node dissection. My surgeon preferred to remove and test my lymph nodes now rather than wait and do it with the mastectomy. I had two nodes removed, and both were clear. Unfortunately, I ended up a few weeks later, back in hospital with an infection.'

'How did that feel?'

'Awful. I felt good for the week following my dissection, but then I started to feel unwell. The week before Easter, I returned to my surgeon's office, who said everything looked fine. Easter Monday and that night pus started to ooze from my wound. It was around 8.00 pm. My partner took me to the local emergency department, and I ended up staying for six nights. The first night they manually expressed the pus from my wound, which was the worst thing ever. Later, I was told to never let them do that again. In the end, I needed to have an ultrasound guided aspiration to fully drain the infection and then antibiotics. What was also a nuisance is that this was the time I was scheduled to have my port put in, but that date has now been moved to next month.'

'So you don't have your port yet, but you have started chemotherapy? How is that going?'

'That's right. I actually started chemo the same week as I started to feel unwell with my infection. Chemo is every three weeks, so I spent a lot of time after my first chemo in bed or in hospital. I had my second dose of chemotherapy two weeks ago. The first week following was awful, and I felt really bad. Nauseous, with no energy, and everything tasted terrible. It's now the end of my second week and I'm feeling a lot better. Next week is my third week and I am hoping to feel normal. Just in time for it all to start again.'

Talking a little more and I discover that breast cancer is not the only illness Kelly is currently dealing with.

'In 2015, I was diagnosed with psoriatic arthritis (a type of inflammatory arthritis), then in 2022, fibromyalgia, which is basically pain throughout your whole body. I was on some heavy medication, which my surgeon has taken me off for the time being. Apparently, breast cancer and chemotherapy supersedes these. I'm also wearing a sleeve as my dissection has caused some mild lymphoedema. At the moment, my left arm is about 1.5-2 cm bigger than my right arm.'

'So after chemo, surgery?'

'Yes. I'm booked to see my specialist again in late August and will most likely be having my mastectomy in September.'

'Will you be having reconstruction?'

'I'm not sure, but I don't think so. I'm fine with being flat and I don't really want any more operations. I think I would like a double mastectomy, although being public, I am not sure if I am eligible.'

'I am not sure either,' I answer. 'But I would push for a double if I could. I think it makes it easier if both breasts are removed.'

'That's what I have also been told, so I'm going to look into it more.'

Like I have with each of my interviews, I ask Kelly if she has learnt anything from her journey so far. I know she has not long begun it, but Kelly already has a great answer.

'I find I'm a lot calmer now. Facing your mortality, things are not worth worrying about anymore. I've come up with a saying, "No expectations, no disappointments." I find myself thinking and saying this often and it really helps.'

'I know you're only three months into your diagnosis, but is there anything you have learnt that would help someone else who is just finding out they have breast cancer?'

'I have found the *Women's Cancer Support - GC* group invaluable. So I would suggest to anyone just diagnosed to find a good support group. Maybe even a cancer mentor if they can. Someone who has gone through this same journey and can offer help and guidance. I would also suggest you take someone to your appointments and to write everything down. It would be good if they gave you a kit or something that contains all the information you will need because there is such a lot to learn.'

'You're not the only person who has said an information kit would be good,' I laugh.

'A friend bought me a gift basket full of items like lip balm, aloe vera toothpaste, a thermometer, blanket, notepad, and books. She doesn't have breast cancer, she has multiple sclerosis, so she knows the system. Knows what someone going through life-changing treatment will need. I had no idea. So, it would be good to have a kit that has a list of things that will be handy so you can be prepared. I would also think about looking at your health and taking natural therapies. My brother-in-law was diagnosed with terminal melanoma and so he put me onto his naturopath, who he thinks, helped saved his life with her treatments. Currently, she has prescribed for me a good probiotic, PEA, vitamin D and something else which I can't remember at the moment.'

'So last question. Is there anything you would like someone who does not have breast cancer to know?'

'That's a hard question,' Kelly ponders for a moment or two. 'But what comes to mind is that with all the great positive press out there about breast cancer, how we get told if you are going to get a cancer, then it's good that it is breast cancer as so much research has gone into it over the years, that it takes away from just how serious a breast cancer diagnosis actually is. People expect me to feel glad that it's breast cancer and not another cancer like ovarian or something, but I'm not glad. They don't realise how sick we can feel. How scared. It was only meeting up with other breast cancer survivors that I could finally acknowledge that this is really serious, that I don't have to answer "good" every time someone asks me how I am feeling. People without breast cancer don't want to hear that you're feeling sick or tired or whatever. I've even felt guilty if I have tried to tell them the truth about how I feel. They just don't want to hear it. So I would tell someone without breast cancer to not tell me it is good it's breast cancer, and to be ready if I tell them how I am really feeling.'

Addendum

Computerized tomography or CT Scans - Unlike an MRI which is better at detecting soft tissue damage, CT scans are better for showing bone and joint issues. Using a series of x-rays, they are combined to build a 2D or 3D image of the inside of your body. They are quick and painless.

CHAPTER
26

Oxana-Invasive Ductal ER Positive Stage 4

———————

IT'S AN ABSOLUTELY GORGEOUS AUTUMN morning when I meet with 46-year-old Russian ex-pat Oxana in the charismatic town of Bangalow. We are sitting in a little outdoor café, gravel crunches crisply underfoot, the smell of great coffee permeates the air and overhead, the sky is the most incredible Mediterranean blue. I'm excited to be here because I think Oxana's story is going to be one of the most memorable, probably the most unique of all the stories I have garnered so far. Before I explain why I expect this, I'll give a rundown on Oxana's initial diagnosis.

Like many others, Oxana had breast lumps. 'For years I had cysts in my breasts and over time I could feel them growing. But what tricked me is that I had them in both breasts, and both were growing simultaneously. So my breasts were getting bigger and perkier, but it was happening in both breasts, so while I was surprised, I didn't think it was anything serious. Cancer doesn't occur in both breasts, hey? I had also gone through a few years of upheaval, so my health came second.'

The years of upheaval Oxana refers to are first a major move from Sydney to the country, then a change in career closely followed by the closure of a business, and finally, her mother's death.

'I used to be a financial advisor in Sydney. After years of living the high-flying lifestyle, about five years ago, I moved to a tiny country town where I had my mortgage broking business. One day, I decided I had had enough of finance, and that I would do something else. I would open my own Russian dumpling business (Oxana moved from Russia to Australia 22 years ago to study IT at university). No one else in Australia was doing this and so I sold my mortgage broking business and opened a dumpling shop called *From Russia with Love*. But then there was a war.' At this, Oxana stops and gives a huge shout of laughter. 'A war! And before that Covid and lockdowns. So, I had to close my shop and just rely on my online business. Then my mum in Russia gets Covid and thirty days later, she dies. What all this does is it makes me stress. So much stress and worry. And behind all this, both of my boobs are growing, and I am ignoring them until one day they get really red and painful. That's when I know to take myself to a doctor.'

This was in December 2021 and after blood tests, biopsies, and an ultrasound, Oxana returns to her doctor mid-January 2022 to receive her results.

'They tell me it's stage 4, ER-positive breast cancer. I think they said ductal, but after hearing it was stage 4, nothing else really mattered. It was in both breasts and my lungs, and while they didn't see it then, a short time later they found it in my bones and in my spine and they told me I was incurable.'

'Did they offer you any treatment?'

'Because it was ER positive, straight away, they put me on Verzenio the same drug as you, but at stage 4 they don't cut you, so, no mastectomy. At stage 4, they leave you to your own devices. They say "well, it's escaped, so we'll just learn to prolong your life. To manage it". They also straight away put me into menopause with injections and they put me on letrozole to block my hormones.'

For eight months, Oxana tells me, she took her Verzenio, her letrozole and continued with the injections that forced her into menopause. 'At first, the lumps started reducing but then I got more spots on my spine, my neck, it went to the pelvic floor. I kept telling the doctors something was not right. It shouldn't still be growing because I had also completely changed my life.'

By completely changing her life, Oxana is referring to her diet, starting with juicing and cutting out sugar; she also went fully vegan and stopped drinking alcohol. Her treatments, she regularly undertook Vitamin C infusions and hypothermia treatment, and her adoption of alternative medications and supplements.

'My partner had found Jane McLelland's book months ago, and I had read it, but it was confusing, so it just sat on my bedside table. Then, about the same time as I was telling the doctors that something was wrong, that nothing was working, I reread Jane's book, learnt about her protocol, the use of off label drugs and I decided that this was it. This was going to save me. This is how I am going to stay alive.'

Oxana doesn't need to tell me the next part of her story, because I already know it. I learnt it via a *Facebook* post she made and is how I first became aware of her. It's why earlier, I said that hers was probably one of the most unique stories I had come across.

Briefly, in January 2023 Oxana had posted on the Jane McLelland *Facebook* site that 12 months earlier she had been diagnosed with stage 4 breast cancer, had metastases to lungs, bones, spine, and skin and after months of declining health and few options from her doctors, had decided to try Jane's protocol. The problem, Oxana had posted, was that Jane's recommended drugs (metformin, doxycycline, atorvastatin and mebendazole), were nearly impossible to get in Australia. Very few doctors would prescribe them. Desperate, Oxana had asked her sisters still living in Russia to obtain them for her. She knew you could get them over the counter in Russia, which they did. Oxana then met her sisters in Turkey and, armed with two enormous boxes of meds, returned home to Australia. Oxana's *Facebook* post had then described how, along with a change in her traditional treatment, and just two months after commencing Jane's protocol, all evidence of her cancer had completely disappeared. It was an incredible story made even more fascinating to me when I learnt Oxana lived close by. I knew I had to meet with her.

Today, I learn a little more of the story.

About a month after Oxana began Jane's protocol, she also finally convinced her doctors to take another biopsy of her cancer. As she said, she had been arguing with them for months, trying to convince them that something was not right. That, because of the changes she had introduced into her lifestyle along with taking their prescribed medication, her cancer shouldn't be getting worse so quickly.

'Finally they said yes, they would retest. It had metastasised to my skin, so they could easily obtain a sample. And I was right. Something was wrong. The test came back HER2 positive with no evidence of ER positive at all. The doctors were shocked. They had been treating me for the wrong type of cancer all along.'

Following this new diagnosis and still on Jane's protocol, Oxana immediately started chemotherapy, where, by session five, around October-November 2022, her cancer had completely disappeared.

'I don't know if it was the chemotherapy or Jane's drugs, but I had an 8 cm tumour and now it had completely gone. As had all the spots on my spine and in my lungs. The doctors couldn't believe it and they asked if I wanted to stop chemo, which I did. There was no cancer left in my body for the chemotherapy to act on. I didn't want to keep poisoning myself and the doctors were telling me that this was as good as it gets.'

While Oxana discontinued chemotherapy, she continued receiving her triweekly injections of Herceptin, a targeted anticancer drug and the primary treatment for HER2 positive cancers, and she continued following Jane's protocol.

'They call being on Herceptin "maintenance", and it was wonderful. I kept thinking, is this it? I just keep taking this and I am cured? But then,' here Oxana pauses before taking a deep breath. 'The fear, the anxiety started. I don't know where it came from, but I started going from a few panic attacks a week to one every day. I kept thinking, will it come back? Will it come back? I started taking Xanax. The worst-case scenario with HER2 cancer is that the Herceptin will stop working.' Oxana pauses again, before giving another shout of laughter, 'and that's what happened to me.'

February 2023 and Oxana knows that something is wrong, that the Herceptin has failed by the huge wedge-shaped lump she could feel growing in her right breast and the skin metastases reoccurring on her left.

'In one month, my lump grew by 6 cm and so I knew it was back. And after more ultrasounds and biopsies, they told me it had "broken through the Herceptin." My oncologist was devastated, and I felt like I had to console him.' Another bark of laughter, although it fades with her next sentence. 'They also told me that the medium survival rate was five years.'

'What's interesting,' I say. 'Is that by still having your breasts, by still being able to feel lumps in them, you could tell that your cancer had returned. They are like a barometer to your cancer.'

'Yes. And I also know my body. I could feel them growing and I knew that these new lumps were not good. But,' she continues, 'I don't think it was because the Herceptin stopped working that caused my cancer to return, I think it was all in here,' and she points to her head.

'Over the last year, I had changed everything, my diet, my lifestyle, everything. The doctors had me on the right drugs, so it shouldn't have come back. But for the past few years, I had lived in fear. Fear about my mum, my son, the business. Always something, some problem, and then the fear that my cancer would come back. And boom, in February it comes back.'

Following this second occurrence, Oxana immediately recommences chemotherapy, seven more rounds of Taxol to finish the regime she started last time. She's still undergoing this as we speak. She has also reread Jane's book a third time, introduced even more supplements into her diet and, convinced her cancer is mainly fear driven, is speaking with shamans and psychotherapists to try to help her cope. In the next day or so, she will be meeting with someone who will be talking to her about psychedelics to ascertain whether taking these is an option. As Oxana says, she has to try everything.

Like I have with everyone, I ask Oxana if she has learnt anything from this journey.

'It's been a horrible experience.' She surprises me with. 'But I am glad that I have had it. I'm a different person now. I used to say things like, I hate this life, but now I have completely changed, completely cleansed myself. I have got rid of all the bitterness. I'm much stronger and my relationship with my partner and son is also much stronger now.'

'You've had to deal with a lot,' I continue. 'Is there anything you could share with those newly diagnosed that may help them with their journey?'

'Don't go looking or reading about other people's stories' she tells me instantly. 'I used to watch heaps of videos about people with stage 4 and other cancers on *Instagram* and other social media platforms. They are not good for you. You see people slowly dying and it messes with you. They don't help you at all. I would also say number one, change your brain and change your lifestyle. And don't give up if they tell you, it's stage 4 or incurable. I hate that word–incurable. I am going to beat this. It went away once and it will again. And remember, life is in your hands. Only you can save yourself.'

Finally, I ask if she has anything to tell those without cancer. Any advice?

'That's my girlfriends,' she laughs. 'I watch them drinking and I know it's not good for them. When my mum died, I started drinking a lot. My lifestyle as a financial advisor also meant I drank a lot. I used to look at myself drinking and think, what will stop you drinking so much Oxana? I knew it wasn't good for me. So, I am now telling my girlfriends, girls, tame it. And be happy with little. That's what cancer teaches you. I never used to say, be happy. But now I say it out loud, be happy. Life is amazing. Love it.'

It's a few days later that I put Oxana's story to paper. Sitting here, thinking of her, remembering her lovely, vivacious face as she tells me she hasn't finished with life yet, that she just needs to rework the chapter concerning her brain and then she will be fine, I'm so scared for her but also so impressed. I know she still has a really rough road ahead, but I feel if anyone is strong and capable enough to traverse it, then Oxana is.

Addendum

Alternative Therapies - A diagnosis of breast cancer means you will be led down the mainstream medical path. In order to support your journey you may wish to investigate alternative therapies such as massage, homeopathy, acupuncture, Chinese medicine, aromatherapy, chiropractic, psychotherapists and many others.

CHAPTER

27

Karen-Papillary Carcinoma Hormone Positive Stage 2

———— ◦◦◦ ————

FLASHBACK TO OCTOBER 2022 - I have just finished radiation, have discarded my mask, and have started to reintegrate back into the real world. Reintegration means I can finally attend one of the monthly lunches organised by the *Women's Cancer Support - GC* group. It's held at a riverside café and overjoyed that I can finally interact face to face with others travelling this same journey, I happily trade stories and make new acquaintances. Two of these acquaintances, Karen and Denise, I meet with again over the following months and when it's time to obtain stories for this book; I approach them both. Denise, diagnosed stage 4 from the outset, is reluctant to meet with me. Her cancer has progressively worsened, and she is not sure if she is up to it. Karen is happy to oblige, which I am grateful for because Karen's cancer is a little different.

In May 2021, aged 56, Karen had her annual mammogram at Breast Screen Australia. With breasts containing cysts and microcalcifications (calcium deposits frequently associated with premalignant lesions) detected in 2018, annual mammograms were a must.

'I had my mammogram in 2018, where they detected the microcalcifications. My 2019 test came back all clear. I missed my 2020 test because of Covid and the death of my mum, then in May 2021, Breast Screen detected something new.'

Further testing revealed that Karen had papillary carcinoma, a rare form of breast cancer that usually has an excellent outcome and is characterised by its unique finger, or 'cottage cheese' shaped appearance as Karen describes it.

'98% of papillary carcinoma cases,' Karen tells me. 'Have a great outlook and generally only need a lumpectomy and maybe some radiation. This was recommended for me initially. Unfortunately, further testing showed that I fell into the 2% of cases without such a good outlook. Mine was invasive papillary carcinoma which has a higher rate of reoccurrence and at the very least, I was advised to have a double mastectomy.'

Late June 2021, Karen has her double mastectomy with the resulting pathology showing her cancer to be stage 2, grade 2, ER and PR positive with no lymph node involvement. Like me, Karen's oncologist also performs a 15-year survival Predict Test.

'My results came back. I had a 76% survival rate of living for 15 more years with surgery alone. Chemotherapy only added another 2.9%. Based on these figures, I decided not to do chemotherapy.'

'Your cancer was ER and PR positive, so what about hormone therapy?' I ask.

'My oncologist prescribed letrozole, which I took for a few months, until October 2021, then I changed to tamoxifen.'

'Why was that?'

'Letrozole was creating havoc with my body. Lots of muscle and joint pain. And I kept putting on weight.'

'And the tamoxifen, are you still on it?'

'I was so scared of the side effects of the tamoxifen, that I took it, but it was a bit hit and miss.'

'So, you had your double mastectomy back in June 2021, then in consultation with your oncologist chose not to have chemotherapy due to the low percentage it added to your overall survival rate. Did anything happen after that?'

'2022 turned out to be a really stressful year. In February, my two-year-old granddaughter came for a visit, and 16 months later, I still have her. Her mother just went awol. She was into drugs, prostitution, and she just took off. I had been working full time as a logistics leader at a local distillery, but suddenly I had a two-year-old to look after. Childcare was going to cost $472 per week, and because this hadn't gone through the courts, we couldn't access childcare assistance. The financial and emotional stress was huge. We also had the floods. I think I had a bit of a mental health breakdown. I just couldn't do it all, so I had to give up work.'

Karen resigned her position in March 2022 and, because she had leave owing to her, doesn't technically finish up until 28 April 2022.

'A week later, on 4 May, I noticed a small hard lump above the scar on my right breast and I just got that sick feeling straight away.'

'What happened then?'

'My GP referred me for an ultrasound and a biopsy, which came back positive for malignant recurrent breast carcinoma, grade 2. I ended up having more surgery where they removed most of my pectoral major muscle. They nearly ring-barked me,' Karen laughs.

'And after your surgery?'

'Pathology showed this cancer to be highly ER and PR positive, even more than last time, so I was again prescribed tamoxifen. I also underwent 15 sessions of radiation. I finished radiation in early August 2022, and I have been sick with colds ever since.'

'So, you're still on tamoxifen, anything else? Did you try supplements or change your diet?'

'No, I haven't changed my diet. I did the tamoxifen from October until about February this year, but it's been a real struggle mentally. I just can't tolerate it and find it a real downer. I've also gained 8 kilos. I've had to go off it again although I am on medication now for high blood pressure, high cholesterol, my heart and also antidepressants. I never had to take any medication before breast cancer, now I am on four.'

Listening to Karen and it's obvious that her journey has been a tough one. Finding herself in the minority group for a cancer that usually has an excellent prognosis. Unexpectedly finding herself having to take on the responsibility of looking after a two-year-old at an age and time when she should have been concentrating on herself. Having to give up a job she loved. Losing her mother. Having to worry about a drug addicted daughter.

'I've been under a bit more stress lately as my daughter has started reaching back. It's been terrifying me. My granddaughter is doing really well. She's in a great environment, attending day care, having dance lessons, swimming. She's happy. I wouldn't be so concerned if my daughter was getting herself together, getting the proper support she needs, but she isn't. She thinks she's fine, but she's not. I recently got a letter addressed to her from the magistrates' courts asking her to appear. There were 16 charges, four were criminal charges, six drug related and five concerning prostitution. I see only three outcomes for her, really. She will get murdered, or she will commit suicide, like her ex-partner, the father of my granddaughter did, or she'll go to jail.'

'Do you ever blame stress for your cancer reoccurrence?' I question.

'Oh definitely. I definitely think it has a lot to do with stress. I am now on anti-depressants; I've been on them for six months, but I feel they are not as effective as they were initially. I've also noticed some new lumps just above the scar on my left side. I really hope they are nothing, just scar tissue, but I don't think so.'

'Are you getting them looked at?'

'I had an appointment for April this year, but because I had a cold, they wouldn't see me. Now I can't get another breast appointment until February next year.'

'Next year, in nine months' time?'

'Yes, February 2024. I've been trying to access an alternative breast specialist, but they are all too busy.'

I'm stunned that someone who has already gone through a cancer reoccurrence cannot get a new appointment for what could be a second reoccurrence. While searching for ladies to interview for this book, I had perceived there were a lot of breast cancer cases around, I just hadn't realised how many. I also had given little thought to the effect all these diagnoses could have on our health care systems. I know Karen is going through the public hospital system and it's a shocking wake up call to see just how stretched, how fragile it actually is.

'It's almost like there is a breast cancer epidemic,' I say in mystification. 'And the system isn't ready.'

As always, I finish our interview with the three questions I ask all these incredible warriors.

'Have you learnt anything from your breast cancer journey?'

Karen takes a long pause before answering me.

'I think this journey has been interrupted by having a now three-year-old. It's taken the focus away from myself. It hasn't been life changing, it's just been a pain in the arse. I have learnt there is no perfect science now. I didn't have chemotherapy after my initial diagnosis. It was supposed to only add a 2.9% increase to my survival rate. Maybe I should have. Also, to trust your gut. With my reoccurrence, the radiologist kept saying it was only a seroma (a pocket of clear fluid under the skin), and they tried to drain it. I knew it was solid, but they kept trying to suck it out, which could lead to tracking, you know, whereby pulling the needle through spreads the cancer cells. I have also learnt that there are a lot of us going through this and there are others worse than me. Like Denise, she's my age, just 58. I visited her in hospital on Tuesday and she is not doing well. She's ready to go.'

Hearing about Denise is a sobering reality check to our conversation, and I take a moment before asking my next question.

'Ok, so, if there was someone else coming along, someone newly diagnosed, is there something you would want them to know? Any treatment tricks. Something you may have learnt?'

'That's hard. There are so many of us and everyone's journey is different. I know some ladies don't want to know any of the technical stuff. Some are just oblivious and couldn't even tell you what type of breast cancer they have. I need to know. I think it's important to know what type it is and what's going on with your own body.'

'Ok, so that was for someone newly diagnosed. What about someone without cancer? Is there anything you would want them to know?'

'You know, I struggle with my body image now. I've put on weight, I used to go swimming, was always active, now I'm not. So maybe I would say, have some compassion. I've had a few insensitive friends. One has had boob job after boob job, she says she can't lose her breasts as she wouldn't be feminine. I had no choice but to have both of my boobs cut off; I just find things like this really insensitive, really hard. I'm also really open. I don't mind talking about my breast cancer, so I like it when people ask.'

'I know what you mean,' I tell her. 'But people don't want to talk about it. I had lunch with a couple of friends recently. Neither of them referred to my cancer at all. Nothing. Cancer is the biggest thing in my life at the moment. You would have thought they would have mentioned it. If I had bought a house or had a baby, it would have been mentioned. Why not cancer?'

It's been one of the most difficult of all my interviews so far. Talking with her, I can tell that this journey has really taken it out of Karen. She looks stressed, exhausted, nearly defeated. It's not helped when a text arrives as we prepare to leave.

'It's from Denise's son,' she tells me sadly. 'Denise passed away 20 minutes ago.'

Addendum

Hormone Therapy - Also known as hormone treatment or endocrine therapy, its aim is to slow or stop the growth of hormone-sensitive tumours by blocking the body's ability to produce hormones. There are different types of hormone therapies (tamoxifen, aromatase inhibitors, ovarian suppression) and what you will be prescribed (if any) depends on your age, breast cancer type, and whether you have reached menopause.

CHAPTER
28

Justine-Invasive Ductal Hormone Positive Stage 4

———❦———

I'VE BEEN INTERVIEWING LADIES FOR over a month now, usually meeting in a café somewhere and over a cuppa, obtaining their incredible stories. But I've yet to come across a really good news story. A story that not only provides hope, but a story that inspires and leaves you determined to try even harder to beat this insidious disease. This changes when I meet Justine, a true warrior if I have ever met one.

November 2017- and 47-year-old Justine, a resident of Mudgee, a regional town in central western New South Wales, pops along to the mobile breast screening van that's making its annual visit to the city. She's been vigilant since the age of 40 about obtaining regular mammograms after watching her mother twice fight the disease. Unlike previous visits, this time her mammogram picks up an abnormality and, following a second mammogram, an ultrasound and a biopsy, a diagnosis of invasive ductal carcinoma stage 2, ER and PR positive, is made.

'These follow-up tests,' Justine tells me, 'were conducted in Dubbo where Breast Screen NSW has their regional office. A drive of about an hour and 20 minutes from where I lived. As soon as I heard my results, I knew exactly what I wanted. I had seen my mother go through breast cancer twice. I had a plan.'

What Justine wants is a double mastectomy. 'I wanted both breasts gone. I didn't care. I just wanted them both off. But my surgeon recommended just the single in order to save the other nipple. Afterwards, I would do my treatment. He said I was fit and strong, therefore they could hit me hard with the chemo and I would be done. Because my lymph nodes were clear, I wouldn't need to undergo radiation.'

On 15 December 2017, Justine makes the hour and a half journey to the regional city of Bathurst, where she undergoes her single mastectomy; chemotherapy will begin in the new year.

'I had a holiday booked for January 2018. I was to go on holiday, then start chemo on my return. Before I went on holidays however, and before I began chemotherapy, my doctor recommended a routine PET, CT and bone scan. So, it was another hour and 30-minute drive back to Bathurst to do them. When the radiologist was doing the bone scan, it was funny,' Justine laughs. 'She did the scan, and I had finished, then she comes back out saying she would just like to do one more scan of my head. Later, I'm telling my daughter about it and laughing and being smart, saying I probably have a brain tumour or something.'

The following week and Justine hears nothing and so she goes on her holiday, where two days in, she retrieves a phone message left on her phone by her doctor's office.

'It says there is a problem with my scans and to phone them,' she tells me. 'Who leaves a message like that?'

The problem, it turns out, is that Justine's bone scan had 'lit up like a Christmas tree.' It showed her breast cancer having metastasised to many of her bones. It was in her thighs, her skull, her spine, sternum, ribs and her hips were covered in it. 'Unbelievably, it wasn't in any of my organs. Just everywhere in my bones.' Justine was now stage 4.

'So, being stage 4 would mean a new treatment plan?' I question. 'What was recommended now?'

'There would be no chemo now. My doctor told me it would be a waste of time. There was a new trial drug out–Ribociclib (like abemaciclib, Ribociclib is a CDK 4/6 inhibitor that targets the proteins that allow cancer cells to divide and grow), which he put me on. I was also prescribed the hormone blocker exemestane and given Zolodex (an estrogen suppressor) injections every 28 days.'

'That was the traditional conventional treatment pathway,' I say. 'How about alternative treatments? Did you search these out?'

It's Justine's response to this, that really sets her aside, makes her a genuine leader, a real inspiration for non-conventional cancer treatment methods. The reason I leave this interview determined to do better with my own cancer fight.

'After my first diagnosis, when I was diagnosed stage 2, I did research different cancer treatments, and I had discovered a holistic functional medicine practitioner living on the Gold Coast, her name was Manuela (this is the same Manuela I had consulted). But it wasn't until I was diagnosed with stage 4 that I contacted her and over zoom, devised a secondary plan to be done in conjunction with my other treatments. At the same time, I was also doing a lot of research online and reading a lot of different books. I followed the *Breast Cancer Conqueror*; read *Chris Beat Cancer*; watched the *Truth about Cancer* documentary; read Nasha Winters' book *The Metabolic Approach to Cancer* which advocates a ketogenic diet. Prior to reading Nasha's book, I had dabbled with keto for weight loss, but following my diagnosis, I said to myself, 'I need to get serious'. I had read a lot about keto, done a lot of research. There's a lot of scientifically proven evidence that keto kills cancer and so I went keto.'

Going keto eventuates to Justine changing her diet completely. From a high fat, high-sugar diet Justine eliminated and continues to do so, most carbohydrates and introduced moderate fats and proteins. 'Cancer feeds off sugar and so I had to starve the cancer by lowering my sugar enough that it created an environment it couldn't live in. To enter ketosis.'

At the same time, Justine turned to a keto diet, she was also working with Manuela, following her recommendations whilst taking the supplements she recommended.

'So a change in diet and supplements. Was there anything else you did?'

'I also started taking cannabis oil. I am scripted for cannabis, which means I meet certain criteria and, after applying to Queensland Health for a script, can get it from a company in Brisbane called Plant Med, rather than illegally from Nimbin. I also use a lot of essential oils which I get from a company called Doterra.'

'Essential oils. What do you do with them?'

'Lots of things,' Justine laughs. 'I inhale them, rub them, take them orally, use them in my cooking. And I detoxed everything.'

'Like your house?'

'Yes. I try not to use any chemicals at all now. I changed my makeup, my shampoo, my toothpaste, my cleaning products, laundry powder. As many things as I could.'

'As an aside and for my own personal curiosity, can you recommend a deodorant and a make-up?'

'I use Inika organic make-up. It lasts really well and the Eco store laundry powder. I've tried loads of different deodorants. I think the cannabis oil gives me bad body odour, so I'm always aware of it. Currently, I'm using a rose one from the Giant Chemist. I can't remember the name, but it lasts all day. I love the Giant Chemist. They have heaps of great stuff.'

All of this occurs in 2018 and apart from a move to the Gold Coast in 2019, 'We moved for medical reasons, really. I just didn't want to have to continue driving for hours to attend appointments,' Justine continues with her new lifestyle. She also continued to have annual PET scans. 'Every scan started showing a reduction in my bone mets with no new growths,' until, in August 2021, Justine is given the extraordinary news that there is no evidence of disease anywhere. Her cancer has completely disappeared. She has defeated it.

'It had totally gone?' I reiterate in awe. 'Totally disappeared? That's incredible. And is this still the case two years on?'

'Yes. Although I am due for my latest scan now. My new oncologist keeps advising me not to keep having them, that I don't need to keep subjecting myself to so much radiation—but I need to for my own sanity. I also decided to have a breast reconstruction last year. I had to think long and hard about whether I wanted to subject my body to so much stress, but in the end, it was worth it.'

Justine's news that, from having bones absolutely riddled with cancer, she is now free of the disease, is so unusual, so inspiring, that I need to take a moment to reflect. I've talked to other stage 4 warriors whose cancer disappeared, but it came back. The major difference between Justine and these others is that Justine really went all out. She completely changed her mindset, her eating habits, her living habits, her environment. It's hard to believe that doing this could cause total expulsion of all cancer, but here she is, living proof that it worked.

'So, a question I ask everyone.' I eventually continue. 'I know it's pretty obvious, but is there anything you have learnt from this journey?'

'Everything happens for a reason,' Justine replies. 'I think this was a real wake-up call. I have had to really give thought to what caused this, my cancer, what lead me down this path. I know it was my diet. I was always a fit and healthy person. I did ironman triathlons, cross-fit six times a week, but we always thought that to stay skinny you had to follow a low-fat diet which we did. But when they remove the fat from something, they replace it with sugar, so really, we were eating a very high-sugar diet. So I have learnt to educate myself on what I eat.'

'Which looks to have worked,' I smile. 'Again, maybe obvious, but there are a lot of newly diagnosed ladies out there. Is there anything you could share with them? Any tricks?'

'I can't stress enough to look at their diet. Read Dr Gundry's *Diet Evolution* book. Be the master of their own disease. So many out there just rely on a magic pill to fix everything. My father, who had prostate cancer, did that. He wasn't prepared to change. I've had people who see me eat come up and say, "I don't know how you do it." And I'm thinking, what? You couldn't give up some sugar in order to save your life? And exercise. It's been proven that exercise helps with chemotherapy, makes it work better. This goes for everything. They must exercise.'

'I agree. Exercise definitely got me through chemo and continues to do so today. This last question is for those without cancer. Is there anything you want to say to them? Anything you would like them to know?'

'Prevention is better than cure. Learn how to prevent it. My daughter is studying to become a dietician. She is educating herself on prevention. I've had to re-educate myself. I've done a ketogenic nutrition course. I've done my yoga training. I am a qualified health coach and currently nearly finished my mindfulness meditation course. I've done most of this after diagnosis.'

It's been an incredible interview, and it's hard ending it. I can't help but feel slightly in awe of Justine. There are few people who would be strong enough to change their way of life completely and permanently. To learn new skills. To re-educate themselves. To basically become a different person, a true survivor. That she has been so incredibly successful makes her story remarkable. Maybe a lesson for us all.

Addendum

Coffee enemas - Although not generally supported by mainstream medical practitioners, integrative doctors promote coffee enemas to detoxify the liver and remove waste from the body. I ended up purchasing a simple enema kit from *Amazon* and use it once or twice a week. Using organic coffee and filtered water, the process is simple and cleansing.

CHAPTER

29

Julie-Invasive Ductal Hormone Positive Stage 4

———— ⌇ ————

I'VE JUST SPENT THE PAST 18 months implementing different strategies to fight off my cancer. I've become vegetarian, eliminated nearly all dairy and alcohol, considered going keto, drastically reduced my sugar and carbohydrate intakes. I've detoxed my house, changed my toothpaste, and then I meet Julie. A 20-year cancer survivor who utterly and decisively blows every assumption I have made about the behaviour of cancer, completely out of the water.

In April 2003, way back when PET scans were virtually unobtainable to everyday Australians and about the time breast cancer was becoming the popular cancer to throw research funds at, then 39-year-old Julie felt a very small lump in her right breast. Concerned, as breast cancer had been diagnosed throughout her family, Julie took herself to a doctor who organised an ultrasound, mammogram, and biopsy. The results came back. Julie had invasive ductal carcinoma, stage or grade 3 (she is unsure which, it was too long ago), ER positive. 'The tumour was 5 cm,' she reflects. 'The size of a small egg.'

Because of her age, back then 39 was considered very young to have breast cancer when most others being diagnosed were well into their 50s and 60s, it was recommended she have a single mastectomy followed by chemotherapy and radiation. Being a hormone positive cancer, Julie was also put on tamoxifen. 'My oncologist told me they would hit it with everything they had.'

Julie spent the rest of 2003 undergoing treatment, which was eight sessions of chemotherapy followed by 36 sessions of radiation, and during this time, she loses her mother. 'Mum had had a heart attack 20 years before, where they only gave her two more years to live. She ended up living another 20. But she was still only 58 when she died.'

It was a hard year, not helped by her husband losing his job and so Julie entered 2004, happy to get a horrible period over with and full of optimism. She had beaten cancer; she was ready to move on. She would even look into having a breast reconstruction.

May 2004, Julie has been meeting with a surgeon discussing reconstruction, when a routine presurgical examination of her remaining breast discloses a new lump. An immediate biopsy is ordered, and Julie is told she once again has breast cancer. Because this is only a tiny lump, they offer her a lumpectomy which she categorically refuses.

'I just said no. I wanted a full mastectomy. I didn't want to have to worry about it returning a third time.'

Again, Julie endures another eight rounds of chemotherapy; fortunately escaping having to have radiation with this diagnosis, and following chemo, undergoes a DIEP flap breast reconstruction. The reconstruction is a success, although it does leave her without nipples, she'll get those sometime down the track.

'So, more chemotherapy; and treatment afterwards? Did you continue with the tamoxifen?'

'No. They took me off tamoxifen and put me onto anastrozole (Arimidex), another, different hormone blocker.'

'How about alternative treatments? Did you consider supplements or anything?'

'I did briefly consider looking at other treatments and I did visit a naturopath, but the problem was, alternative treatment is so costly. We didn't have much money. My husband had lost his job. I couldn't work much.'

'So you pretty much continued your normal lifestyle? Ate the same, no alternative treatment, no supplements?'

'That's right. I was a smoker, so I continued to smoke and still do. I continued drinking and still do. I ate what I wanted and still do. The only thing my stomach could tolerate during my first chemo was coke, so I drank that.'

Determined to get on with her life, Julie spends the rest of 2004 recovering from her treatment and reconstructive surgery, working odd jobs and being a mother to two teenage children.

Early 2005 and pain in her tailbone, sees Julie once again undertaking a bone scan. A small dot is found on her sternum and, incredibly, her medical team ignores it. 'They said it was nothing,' Julie scoffs. Months pass and Julie has another bone scan; what was a small spot on her sternum has now grown to over 6 cm. 'So they did a biopsy, which was quite painful. They had to go in through my chest wall.'

The results of the biopsy come back and, not surprisingly, reveal that Julie's breast cancer has metastasised. 'Although this time, they tell me it's not ER positive but HER2 positive. They also think that last year's cancer may have been HER2 positive as well, but they treated it as estrogen positive like my first cancer. So I had to do another eight rounds of chemotherapy and afterwards they put me on Herceptin, and I also started immunotherapy.'

'Herceptin is used to treat HER2 cancers, isn't it? And immunotherapy. How did you have that?'

'I have it intravenously (via a vein) every three weeks. I'm still on it now, 18 years later.'

'You've had to be treated intravenously every three weeks for the past 18 years. Wow! Is it via a port?'

Julie laughs when I ask this. 'I had a port for my first chemo, which they removed just before my second diagnosis. They had to replace it, but it fell apart in my body. My third port just didn't work, and I got my fourth, the one I still have now, in 2011.'

'So, you spent the greater part of 2005 fighting cancer for a third time? And after that?'

'I just moseyed along, being a mum, getting on with things. I had my nipples reconstructed in 2007 and I continued with the Herceptin, Arimidex and the immunotherapy. Every six months, I would have another bone scan. In 2008, a scan revealed it had spread to my lower spine. This time, they put me on a new chemotherapy drug, Abraxane. My oncologist called me a guinea pig because the drug was new, and I was one of the first to take it.'

'So, your fourth round of chemotherapy? Was this also intravenously or via a tablet?'

'Again intravenously. This time for six months. Since then, I've been having regular bone scans and new spots have appeared on my ribs and on my neck, but my oncologist doesn't want to call them a progression of my cancer because it would mean I would have to come off the Herceptin and that is what has been working the best. Allowing me to have a life.'

'And in the years following. Has anything else happened?'

'In 2013, another bone scan revealed a lesion in my left femur, but it wasn't a concern then. I was working at Coles, continuing with my Herceptin and Arimidex, continuing my usual lifestyle. Then two years later, in 2015, I was at work and had gone out for smoko. As I was walking back inside, I got the most incredible pain in my leg. You know when you just give a yelp of pain, and everyone stares. I just had to lie down on the footpath, and I said to my co-worker, "I think you need to call an ambulance as I am pretty sure my leg has just fractured."'

Julie's leg, it turns out, had fractured. She's taken to hospital where a rod is inserted and for the following few years finds herself pretty much couch bound, crippled by incredible pain. 'It was so intense. Mainly at the fracture site, but in other areas as well. I found myself needing Endone every three hours plus fentanyl patches and regular Panadol osteo. In the end, they had to take the rod out and replace it with another, smaller one, which was a little better. They also took me off the Arimidex and swapped me to Femara (letrozole). It's funny. For years while I was on the Arimidex, I had terrible stomach pain. The moment I switched to Femara, the stomach pain stopped.'

Over the following years, Julie continues having issues with the rod in her leg and is today, early June 2023, still waiting to have another operation which will hopefully fix whatever problem it is that results in her leg causing her so much pain. Although, 'in 2017,' Julie tells me, 'I learnt reiki which I would do religiously. It helped enormously, and I was able to go off all the heavy pain meds. And about eight months ago, probably November 2022, I started using cannabis spray.'

'Cannabis spray? How did you access that and is it working?' I ask.

'It was interesting. Back when I fractured my leg, my oncologist offered to put me on a cannabis trial. At this stage, the trial was for nausea, but I said no. Last year, I went back to him and asked if there were any other trials and while he advised the studies had ended, he could still get me onto cannabis, which he did. I've found that it really helps. Most of my pain has disappeared except for the leg pain. It doesn't help with that.'

As I have been speaking with Julie, what has become obvious is that unlike many other cancer fighters, me included, she hasn't let cancer dictate her lifestyle. We have met at a Chinese restaurant and while I have a plate of frankly boring looking vegetables in front of me, Julie's plate is loaded with some type of gooey sauce covered fried chicken along with fried rice. As she said earlier, she eats what she wants, meat and sugar included. She loves a drink and continues to smoke. She's been this way for the entire time she has had cancer, and she is still alive, nearly 20 years down the track. When I ask her, why does she think this is, how come someone with stage 4 breast cancer can still smoke and drink and live, she gives a loud roar of laughter.

'I have absolutely no idea. Early in my diagnosis, I joined a support group. Unlike me, they ate healthily, took supplements, stopped drinking. And now they are all dead and I'm still here. I've been smoking since the age of 11. Couldn't afford supplements and such. People have come up to me and asked what they should do, what supplements they should take. I just laugh at them and tell them I am not the best person to ask.'

'Maybe it's your tough Kiwi genes,' I grin. 'So apart from eating what you want, do you think you have learnt anything from this journey?'

Again, another peal of laugher. 'I've learnt to not put up with shit from people. I don't tolerate dickheads anymore. I've also learnt that you should do what you want to do although that has been a struggle for me because I haven't had much money. People don't like to employ people with cancer. When I have managed to get work, it's usually by not telling them until later that I have cancer. I've learnt that.'

'So, I have just a few more questions. The first is, is there anything you could share with someone newly diagnosed with breast cancer?'

Julie pauses for quite a while, searching for an answer. 'I don't like to talk to the newly diagnosed girls. I don't like to scare them, so I'm really guarded by what I say. Especially if they have been newly diagnosed with mets. If I had to share anything, it would be that they should always get a second opinion if they are not happy about something. Especially their health care team. That if it doesn't feel right, then change it. Also, live life. Go out and do things. A couple of years ago, I set myself some challenges. I had always wanted to zipline, so I put my leg brace on, took lots of Endone and went and did it. I got my sister to come with me. We had a ball. Then 12 months ago, I went parasailing, again with my sister. I also took one of my oncology nurses as well. We had a few drinks beforehand, and it was the best thing. I would like to do a parachute jump next, but with my leg the way it is, I don't think so. My next challenge will be to get into the water with some whales. Some friends gave me a voucher a while ago to swim with dolphins which I did, so next it's whales.'

'It sounds like you're living your life,' I reply. 'Ok. Now for all those who don't have cancer. Is there anything you would want them to know?'

Again, another pause. 'Don't whinge over minor things. Either say nothing or fix it. If their toe is sore or something. Do something about it.'

Julie's answer to this last question is informative. I suppose it's an answer that only someone who has gone through four rounds of chemotherapy, radiation, countless medications and indescribable pain can give. She's been through so much, had to keep fighting so often, that minor concerns are laughable, not worth thinking about.

Driving home from our meeting, I have to admit that I'm slightly bewildered. My thoughts, in a bit of a turmoil. I'm still trying to fathom how someone who has smoked since they were 11, who drinks, who eats anything and everything, who doesn't take supplements, doesn't use alternative therapies, is still alive 20 years after their initial cancer diagnosis. Many of these choices, through monetary constraints, were forced onto Julie. Maybe it's what has saved her.

Addendum

Cannabis for medicinal purposes – Marijuana, derived from the cannabis family of plants and generally perceived as a recreational drug, is being increasingly recognised as providing benefit to cancer patients. Tetrahydrocannabinol (THC) and cannabidiol (CBD), the two primary active ingredients used in medical application, have been successfully used to treat chemotherapy and cancer side-effects such as pain and nausea. Olivia Newton-John used cannabis oil to alleviate her pain.

CHAPTER

30

Polly-Invasive Ductal HER2 Positive Stage 3

———

IT'S A GLORIOUS AUSTRALIAN WINTER'S day when I meet up with 37-year-old Polly and her cheeky nearly three-year-old daughter, Ayla. Normally challenging attempting anything with a boisterous toddler around, Polly has come prepared, and so while a distracted Ayla happily dances around the café to the music playing on her mum's phone, I get Polly's story. It eventuates to be a wonderful tale of great courage and huge hurdles and it's spoken in a calm, soothing voice that totally belies the storyteller's age. At the end of my interview, I depart thinking that I have probably met one of the bravest, certainly one of the most capable, breast cancer warriors yet.

The year was 2016 and Polly was in the throes of breast-feeding her eldest daughter, 20-month-old Riley, when she noticed a lump on her chest. Situated between her breasts, she thought nothing of it, assuming it was just an accumulation of breast milk, or something connected to her breastfeeding. Fast forward a few months to February 2017 and Polly, after weaning Riley, notices that the lump is still there. Her husband even comments on it, asking what is it and how long has she been aware of it. Still not that concerned—after all Polly is only 31 and breast cancer is an older lady's problem—it's a few more weeks before Polly takes herself to a doctor who organises a biopsy at the local hospital.

'Just a breast biopsy?' I question. 'What about a mammogram or ultrasound?'

'No. Because of my age, it was just a biopsy.'

Two weeks later and Polly returns to the hospital for her biopsy accompanied by Riley.

'My husband worked long hours and all my friends and family live in New Zealand. There was no one to look after Riley, so she ended up coming to all my appointments.' Polly explains in her easy-going manner.

The result of this biopsy warrants a second one and so, a week later, Polly and Riley return to hospital.

'This time, they did a large needle biopsy and blood spurted everywhere.' Polly tells me. 'And Riley is there watching and all she can say is "oh Mumma."'

Another week passes, and it's now mid-April when Polly and Riley make the familiar journey back to hospital where a lovely doctor tells Polly she has invasive ductal carcinoma, stage 3, grade 2, HER2 positive. It's a nasty diagnosis and something Polly wasn't expecting at all.

'I went there thinking it would be a quick appointment to say everything was fine. I had even organised a play date for Riley straight after. So, I'm just sitting there trying to absorb what she is saying, listening to all this medical jargon that doesn't make sense. Riley is just losing it and I'm thinking that we are going to be late for the play date. I think I just sort of zoned out, but then the doctor started speaking Māori to me. She was a Chinese doctor, yet she was speaking Māori, which really calmed me. And then she said something which snapped me out of it. She said, "It's not as if you are going to die or anything, come on." This totally brought me back to reality and so I just asked her what I needed to do, what needed to be done. She said, "It needs to be cut out."'

Cut out, means Polly is offered the choice of a lumpectomy or single mastectomy but because of the position of the tumour on her chest, it's in the middle of her cleavage and a lumpectomy would eliminate the possibility of reconstruction down the track, Polly chooses a right breast mastectomy.

'I then asked when could I have the mastectomy and she said in four days' time if I wanted. So that meant I had to organise everything then and there. I had to go and see the breast care nurses and get mastectomy bras and other stuff. I had to go and see everyone I had to see, fill out all the paperwork, talk to the prep surgery people. I had to phone my husband and tell him the news. I had arrived for my appointment at 8.30 am and didn't leave until 2.30 pm. You can imagine the state of my toddler by then.'

Four days later, on Easter Tuesday, Polly has her mastectomy. Incredibly, a close friend, currently in hospice succumbing to her own breast cancer battle, offers to pay for Polly's mum to fly out from New Zealand and so Polly is not alone.

'So, you had your mastectomy. And the treatment afterwards?' I question.

'I had to return to the hospital the following week where I thought they said I would need just six weeks of chemo, but it was actually six rounds which would take like 18 weeks. Because there was so much involved and I had no support, the really nice doctor who could speak Māori, suggested I go back to New Zealand because following the chemotherapy, I would also need radiation and I would also be on Herceptin for about a year.'

'And is this what you did?'

'I did, but before I returned to New Zealand, my doctor mentioned I may want to think about storing some eggs if I wanted more children. This would need to happen in Australia and before I began chemotherapy. The breast care nurses put me onto a specialist in Brisbane who could do this and the only appointment I could get was at 7 am, so one morning, really early, Riley and I got in the car and drove to Brisbane.' (Brisbane is situated just over an hour north of where Polly lives).

With time tight (it's recommended you commence chemotherapy within four to six weeks of a mastectomy), Polly is immediately started on special IVF drugs which will grow and mature her eggs and early June 2017, returns to the IVF clinic to see if they have developed enough for harvesting and storage.

'We had to return each day for four days and unfortunately, this first round was unsuccessful. They hadn't matured enough. But I had already booked medical appointments in New Zealand, so I ended up quickly flying to New Zealand to meet with my new medical team. I took Riley with me and left her with my mum. My husband was still working, so could not come with me or look after Riley.'

Late June and Polly flies back to Australia alone, where this time her eggs have matured enough for them to be harvested and mixed with her husband's sperm.

'They ended up creating 13 embryos, of which six were of really good quality,' Polly tells me.

Early July 2017 and Polly reunites with Riley in New Zealand (her husband will remain in Australia and continue working), where a port is shortly inserted and where she spends the following five months undertaking chemotherapy and radiation treatment.

'Because chemotherapy turns your eggs into the eggs of a 61-year-old,' Polly tells me. 'They also put me onto Zolodex, a hormone blocker, which put me into early menopause. I also began triweekly Herceptin infusions, which I would continue to take for the following year.'

'How did you go with all of this? Any side effects?'

'I had no problems with chemotherapy or radiation. I did lose my hair, but that was ok. I didn't get any radiation burns, but in January 2018, after I had returned to Australia, I had to stop taking Herceptin for six weeks because of the strain it was putting on my heart. I finished with the Herceptin in September 2018.'

'So that was the end of your active treatment? Did you end up using your frozen eggs?'

'Once I finished treatment completely, I had to return to my doctors for check-ups. At first, it was every three months, then every six, then yearly. Every time I would ask them if it was safe for me to have a baby now or to try for a baby. Each doctor I saw gave me a different answer. My oncologist said wait for five years, meaning I would be 37 before I could have another baby, while my lovely doctor said to just try when I was ready. When I wanted to.'

'And?' I prompt.

'In November 2019, I met with an IVF specialist who did some tests and performed a physical examination. It cost me $300, and he told me to come back in a few weeks to do more tests and to get some blood work done. Not long after this, I started feeling really tired and not that well. I had all the classic cancer symptoms, and I was worried my cancer had returned and so my GP ordered a chest ultrasound for me. On the morning of my ultrasound, my GP did a pregnancy test just to rule that out, and it came back positive. Because I already had an ultrasound booked, they did it on both my chest and my stomach, which confirmed that I was pregnant and that I had been pregnant when I saw the IVF specialist. He just hadn't told me. Ayla was born in July 2020, right into Covid.'

'That's incredible.' I laugh. 'Especially after everything you went through. It must be your tough Kiwi genes.' (I'm seeing a pattern here involving strong ladies originating from New Zealand). 'I sometimes ask if Covid affected treatment. It didn't affect your treatment, but did it affect your pregnancy?'

'It did, but I loved it. It meant I could stay home with both Riley and Ayla. Riley didn't appreciate being home-schooled, but I didn't mind. It meant we didn't have to go anywhere.'

It's taken a while to reach this stage of our conversation and incredibly, Ayla is still fine, still behaving incredibly well. This conduct is no doubt brought about by a babyccino and the promise of a donut on the way home. Even so, I'm impressed. You don't often see toddlers entertaining themselves for nigh on 90 minutes. Knowing I need to wrap our interview up shortly, I quickly ask my usual questions.

'Is there anything in particular you have learnt on this journey? Talking with you, it's obvious that this has been really life changing, but is there anything that stands out to you?'

'Live life in the moment,' Polly replies. 'Create experiences rather than wait for them. Being a young mum with breast cancer, I have also learnt that there is not much information out there for people like me. I was concerned about breast feeding after being on such heavy drugs, whether or not it was safe. I found it really hard to find any information. Likewise, breast feeding with only one boob. I've learnt that it's incredibly hard to find information about things like this. You just have to keep reading, keep searching the internet.'

'Cancer is normally associated with an older age group,' I acknowledge. 'Your searches involved subjects I would never have given thought to. Although,' I ruminate. 'These days breast cancer is appearing to become more and more a younger person's problem as well.'

'Yes. It is. Younger people are being diagnosed, but for now, I'll just have to keep doing my own research,' Polly agrees.

'How about lifestyle changes?' I ask. 'Did you change diet, use supplements or anything like that?'

'I don't like to exercise, but I exercise now. I'm scared not to. I've actually started working in a gym so that I go to the gym. I've also started working in childcare, which helps a lot. Ayla can come with me, so we save having to pay for childcare. My husband has also had to make some lifestyle changes. He is a lot more supportive, and he has had to admit that earlier on, he wasn't always there for me. He is now. He also has a better job. He's become a fly in-fly out worker, so more money, which all helps.'

'And is there anything you would want someone newly diagnosed to know? Any treatment tricks, etc.'

'I would say to just take it all as it comes. Just listen and get it done. My doctor telling me I wasn't going to die really helped me to just deal with it.'

'And for those without cancer. Anything you would want them to know?'

Polly's reply is instant. 'If you ever meet someone with cancer, it's about them, NOT you. We don't want to have to console you when we talk about our illness.'

It's been a memorable interview for many reasons. Polly has undoubtedly been the bravest warrior I have met to date, and it's hard to believe that this gorgeous woman with the beautiful calm voice is also one of the youngest breast cancer fighters I have met. I'm not sure there are many out there who could go through what she has and come out the other end so positive and composed. To fight such a horrible diagnosis while looking after a two-year-old, to jump between two countries for treatment, to leave your husband for months on end, to go through fertility treatment. As I said, a memorable interview.

Addendum

Deep Breath Hold - Administering radiation to the left side of the chest could result in damage to the heart. To mitigate this, patients learn the deep breath hold – a technique whereby taking a deep breath and holding it, moves the heart into a more favourable position. I found it wise to do some practice beforehand.

CHAPTER
31

Bianca-Triple Negative

WHEN I TOLD MY 24-YEAR-OLD daughter that I was off to interview 25-year-old Bianca for this book, she uttered an exclamation of disbelief. Understandable really. People this age don't expect to get breast cancer. It's an older person's disease and something, Bianca advises, completely off their radar. Heck. Most girls her age never even check their breasts for lumps.

Which is fortunate that one day Bianca noticed hers.

It was just seven months ago, in December 2022 and Bianca was enjoying a cruise with her parents, her aunt, uncle and cousins. One morning, while drying herself off after showering, she felt a lump under her left breast. 'It was so noticeable that I wondered how I hadn't noticed it before. I was also feeling a little miserable, like I had a cold or something, so I was thinking, lymph nodes swell when you have a cold, so that must be it. There is no way this lump could have just come out of nowhere.'

Bianca mentions the lump to her mum and as soon as the cruise is finished, they make an appointment to see a doctor.

'Mum was freaking out and automatically assuming the worst, but I was going, mum, I'm 25, it'll just be a cyst or something.'

Bianca's doctor is vigilant, and the same day as her appointment, she undergoes an ultrasound and, two days later, a breast biopsy.

'A few days after my biopsy, my doctor phones to tell me it is a form of breast cancer, but further tests are needed to work out exactly what type.'

More tests eventuate to be a second biopsy, an MRI and a mammogram.

'This was all happening over the Christmas, New Year period, so I had to wait for my results. It was a two week wait, and it was horrendous. Just stressing out waiting.'

On 9 January 2023, Bianca, accompanied by her parents, returns to hospital where she is told she has triple negative breast cancer.

'Did you find out what stage and grade?' I query.

'I didn't. It was all just too overwhelming. There was lymph node involvement as well and while I think he may have said, stage 2 and grade 2, don't quote me on that. I'm not sure.'

'A breast cancer diagnosis is an immense shock for anyone,' I reply. 'But I can't imagine what it's like for a 25-year-old to be told.'

'It was a huge shock and especially for my mum. Breast cancer is not in the family, so we had no idea where it came from. I did genetic testing, but that all came back fine. I have one suspicion, though. I have been on the pill since the age of 13, so maybe that had something to do with it.'

'I've had another lady blame things on the pill as well.'

'I mentioned it to a nurse, and she said, no, it wouldn't have caused it, but just read the pill packet. It says breast cancer could be linked to taking the pill, so who knows?'

'So, one day, out of the blue, you get this horrible diagnosis. What had you been doing beforehand?'

'I'm a filmmaker. I'm a self-employed videographer and was just focusing on my career, really. I actually had plans to go to LA for three months in February this year. I had even bought my ticket just two weeks before my diagnosis. I was super excited about it all and then it all just fizzled out.'

'It can still happen.'

'Exactly. But you know, when I think back, if I had gone then, I probably wouldn't have done anything about my lump. I would have left it until I got back. So there is a positive in everything.'

Hearing Bianca say this really gives me an insight into her personality. I had felt her strength from the confident, cheerful way she had greeted me, but hearing her find positives in what had to be a devastating disappointment, cements just how tough, how capable, she is. I can't help not only admiring her, but really liking her.

'So treatment. What did you have to do?'

'I started with Taxol first. I had to go each week for 12 weeks. It treated me kindly.'

What Bianca means by treating her kindly is that she didn't get many of the awful side-effects that others do, although by week four, she did begin to lose her hair.

'I loved my hair. I had a lot, and it was blue. I think losing it was the worst part of all this. It started coming out in clumps at first, then when I decided to shave it all off, I made it into an event. I invited my family, aunt, uncle and cousins, and my hairdresser shaved it while I filmed it. She didn't just shave it all in one go, but she created different wacky styles as she went along. It was fun and it will be a thing I definitely remember and smile about.'

'Did you consider using a cold cap for your hair and ice socks for your hands and feet?'

'That's the thing. I hadn't heard of these. No one told me. I know now. Joining the *Cancer Support* group has taught me a lot, but at the time, I didn't know. '

'Did you manage to get out much? Meet with your friends?'

'I stayed pretty active, went for walks, played tennis. It was just the work side of things I couldn't do. I record live music which involves mush pits and sweaty crowds. My oncologist was just, no.'

'So, you began Taxol in January, which means you would have finished around the end of April. What did you do next?'

'AC (the Red Devil). Once every three weeks. As I said, Taxol was pretty kind to me, but AC was like, next level brutal. It's not fun at all. My treatment day is on a Friday and so that night, I have pretty severe nausea and then I have really bad reflux for the next week and a half. Nothing gets rid of it, and it gets to the point where I don't want to do anything. But then once that is over, I'm pretty good and back to normal. Then it starts all over again. I've had three sessions so far, and I have had to go to hospital twice.'

'Really, hospital. What for?'

'The first time I was in hospital for five nights with neutropenia sepsis (an infection in those with a low white blood cell count), the second time was because, although I felt fine, my blood tests showed I had this again. I have my final AC tomorrow. I'm hoping I have no problems this time.'

'And afterwards? Will you be having surgery or anything?'

'I'm meeting with my doctor next week to work out the next steps. I had my first follow-up scan, an MRI last week, so I'll find out the results of that. Whether my tumour has shrunk. I'm pretty confident about everything, but there will be surgery of some sort. I think the choice is a double mastectomy with reconstruction or a lumpectomy. Maybe radiation or an oral chemo tablet. I'll do what's recommended.'

Hearing Bianca speak so rationally about maybe having a mastectomy, maybe a lumpectomy, maybe radiation, it's hard to believe I am speaking with a 25-year-old. I've met with numerous cancer fighters on this journey, most more than twice Bianca's age, yet she is coming across as wiser and more positive than many of them. It just seems so unfair that this gorgeous vibrant girl should have to make such awful choices, undergo such toxic treatments at such a young age.

'I mentioned your friends earlier. How did they take the news about your breast cancer?'

'They were blown away at first. Shocked. But now they sometimes come to my treatments with me. We play cards and board games and are the noisy ones in the corner. It's good, as it makes it go so much quicker.'

'Did they run out and get tested for breast cancer?'

'I don't know if anyone has. I think it comes down to a financial thing. They just don't offer mammograms or anything to people our age. But they are definitely more aware.'

'I hadn't thought of that. In Australia, they are only free if you are over 40. There is no incentive for those younger to get tested. That's interesting.' I muse. 'How about lifestyle changes? Did you change your diet, take supplements or anything?'

'I did start eating meat again.'

'Really. I did the opposite.'

'Yes. I had been a vegetarian for four years, but I started craving it and thought, why make it more difficult for myself? I was the only vegetarian at home. I still live with my mum and dad, and it just made it more difficult for everyone preparing something different for me. I wasn't a drinker or a smoker and haven't looked at supplements. I talked to my oncologist about all this, but he said just to stay balanced. I suppose my biggest lifestyle change is that I couldn't work, and that bothered me. I feel like I am seeing everyone else move forward with their lives and I'm just here, waiting to do what I want to do again. But it could be so much worse.'

'You're having a year off.'

'Exactly. I'm having the gap year I never had. Minus the travel.' We both laugh.

'Do you think you have learnt anything from all this?'

'Yes. I feel that as much as all this sucks, it's given me more time to think about what I want to do once this has all passed. What direction I want my life to go. It's made me realise that life is short, and you should do what you want to do and love. So, I have been focusing on music a lot more, which has helped a lot. I want to finish all this feeling positive.'

'So, if there was a person coming along, newly diagnosed with breast cancer, is there anything you would want them to know?'

Bianca takes a moment to answer this question.

'You know, that's so hard, everyone is so different, but I would say to just go with the flow, don't overthink things and don't Google anything. Oh, there is something else,' she cries. 'I wish I had known that 25-year-olds can get breast cancer without having any symptoms or family history. I wish they educated us more about this in school. I mean, we were told about skin cancer, but they don't talk about young people getting breast cancer.'

'That's a pretty powerful answer,' I reply. 'And for someone without breast cancer, is there anything you would want them to know?'

Again, there is a pause.

'I think I would say, if you know someone who has cancer, then don't treat them any differently. I feel like a lot of people feel awkward when talking to someone with cancer. I would say just to treat them how you would normally treat someone. Also, maybe don't tell them they are going to be ok every five minutes because it makes us feel as if we are going to die. My grandma says this a lot. She means well, but the more people say this, the more it freaks me out. I'm aware of how serious the situation is, but I just want to be treated how they used to treat me. I could also say, especially to young people without breast cancer, that you don't need to have big boobs, I don't have any boobs, or a family history, to get breast cancer. There is no criteria, so check yourself. It only takes two minutes, so check yourself and save yourself the pain of having to go through this.'

'Had you been checking yourself?'

'No. I hadn't. There is no information out there, no young people on social media talking about this, which is why I have started putting it out there. I've made a video for people my age to check ourselves, but it's such a private thing. How much do I share? How much don't I share? I don't know, but they need to check themselves.'

'Well, I'll definitely be getting my 24-year-old daughter to look at your video.'

'Good' Bianca replies.

Addendum

General Practitioner – Your GP may have initiated your journey by referring you to a breast specialist. Ensure you pop back to them regularly to keep them updated on your progress. They can provide invaluable ongoing assistance with referrals and medications. Their prescriptions, referral letters, help, will also be required once you have finished active treatment.

Your Breast Surgeon – Will read your initial scans and perform a physical examination. The results of these should dictate what type of surgery, if any, they will perform.

CHAPTER

32

Nicki-Triple Negative Stage 3

———————————

I'VE MENTIONED A FEW TIMES throughout this book that the breast cancer fighters many of us older women feel for the most, are the younger diagnosed ladies, especially those with dependent children. Today, I meet one of the nicest people I have ever met and unfortunately, if there is anyone who could typify this description, then it's Nicki.

Mother to four ranging from nine to twenty-two (the eldest is a stepchild), it was in October 2021, that 36-year-old Nicki noticed that the lymph nodes under her right arm were slightly swollen, somewhat painful. Knowing that she had recently had a Covid vaccine and reassured by media that swollen nodes were a common side effect of the vaccine, Nicki had just brushed it off.

'I remember hearing about Carrie Bickmore on *The Project*. She had been talking about how following their Covid vaccine, a lot of ladies had noticed swollen lymph nodes which had prompted them to go and get checked for breast cancer, but the results were coming back negative. That it was just a normal reaction to the vaccine. So, I ignored it. I called it my Covid pain.'

A month later, November 2021 and the pain is still there, 'I could also feel a slight lump under my arm, but it was right over on the outer edge of my breast. It was painful and when I pushed it, it would move. I had looked up the symptoms of breast cancer and this lump didn't fit with what I had read. Breast cancers don't move. It was more like a swollen lymph node.'

Christmas passes and in late January with the lump still present, still painful, Nicki takes herself to the doctors.

'Even then, my doctor told me she didn't think it was anything to be concerned about. That it was likely just a swollen gland.'

'But she orders you tests?'

'Yes. She sent me for a mammogram and an ultrasound. The mammogram didn't pick up anything, but the ultrasound did.'

What the ultrasound has detected is concerning enough for Nicki's doctor to send her immediately for a breast biopsy and an MRI.

'While they sent me for a biopsy, they pretty much knew from the ultrasound that it was serious.'

Early February 2022 and Nicki learns just how serious. Her biopsy results come back positive for triple negative breast cancer, stage 3 and grade 3. Aggressive and advanced, it's a whisper away from stage 4.

'It's interesting,' Nicki muses. 'I found out later that my lump was 3.5 cm, yet it never showed up on the mammogram. That's scary. Why is that the screening treatment if it so commonly misses things?'

'I'm hearing that a lot,' I agree. 'Do you know if yours was in the duct or in the lobe?'

'I wasn't told. But I was told that I had dense breasts, which makes cancer harder to detect.'

Because chemotherapy is the primary treatment for triple negative breast cancer, Nicki immediately undergoes neo-adjuvant therapy. Surgery will occur down the track.

'So I had a port inserted, which I still have, and then I started on carboplatin and paclitaxel for 20 sessions followed by the Red Devil for 4.'

'I've never heard of carboplatin.'

'I think it's a chemotherapy drug they like to use for triple negative. I would have this one week along with the Taxol, then the following week I would have Taxol and an immunotherapy drug.'

'So you were also on immunotherapy?'

'Yes. It cost me $60,000.'

'$60,000!' I exclaim.

'Yes. I was really lucky that I had a whole lot of friends and community who rallied around and were able to do some pretty amazing fund-raising events so that I could get this treatment.'

'No one's mentioned the cost of this to me before,' I puzzle.

'It depends on what cancer you have. Some cancers are approved for it to be covered on the PBS (pharmaceutical benefit scheme). Actually, in March this year, mine was approved for people with triple negative breast cancer but last year, when I had it, it wasn't. The doctors said that obviously it was a lot of money, but triple negative, stage 3, grade 3, we need to throw everything at it.'

'So you had this at the same time as your chemotherapy? Did you have any problems?'

'I did get Covid twice during my treatment.'

Nicki underwent her treatment pretty well at the exact time I did, March to August 2022. A period when Covid still loomed largely in Australia. While I was dependent free and thus able to isolate myself from most of the outside world, Nicki, with four children, didn't have this luxury. It's not surprising she caught Covid twice.

'What did getting Covid mean for your treatment?'

'I had to push out two of my sessions. That was because I got neutropenia. Where my white blood cells were really low and my body was too weak for chemo. It affected my heart as well. I had started having trouble with my heart after my Covid vaccine. I think they call it an ectopic heartbeat where it beats too fast. Getting Covid made it worse.'

'But you did manage to finish treatment?'

'I finished my chemo but with the immunotherapy, you pay $60,000 and that gives you a certain number of doses, then after that it's free. I was meant to be on it for two years, but I had to stop.'

'Why did you have to stop?'

'Because when I went for my surgery, I had an anaphylactic shock to one of the anaesthetics they gave me.'

Nicki is quite matter of fact when she tells me this, but the story she then relays is anything but.

In August 2022, having finished with chemotherapy (but not immunotherapy as this would run for two years), Nicki is on the operating table, ready to have a double mastectomy. At some stage, they administer her rocuronium, a muscle relaxant, which immediately causes her to go into cardiac arrest.

'My heart stopped beating for nine minutes. They thought they had lost me. Even when they got my heart back, it wasn't a proper rhythm, so I had to get shocked. It took them half an hour to get me back into a proper heart rhythm. My poor husband.'

'He didn't know this was happening, did he?'

'He got a phone call to say that I had had a cardiac arrest, and that they were still trying to stabilise me. That I wasn't out of the woods and that he needed to come to the hospital straight away.'

'Wow. You must have terrified everyone. So, then you woke up?'

'I woke up three days later. They had put me into an induced coma.'

'So when you woke up. Did you have boobs?'

Despite the serious nature of the discussion, both Nicki and I laugh simultaneously at this point. Maybe to lessen the tension.

'Yes, I woke up, and I still had boobs. I was on a ventilator and everyone was really concerned. Because I hadn't had oxygen for so long, they didn't know if I was going to be ok so they were all surprised when I could wiggle my toes and everything. But I woke up, thinking I had just been asleep for surgery. I had no idea of any of this. That this had happened. I was really dazed and confused, and I looked down and was thinking, why do I still have my boobs? Even though they explained everything to me, I couldn't really process it. It took like a day for me to realise what had happened.'

Nicki spends the following week in intensive care, followed by a few days on the ward.

'At some stage, I thought I was having another heart attack. I was getting a lot of pain in my chest, but it turned out to be a broken sternum from when they were doing the CPR on me.'

'Did you still go ahead with your double mastectomy?'

'My immunologist, oncologist, anaesthetist, the entire team, got together for a consult. My immunologist told me that usually they wouldn't put someone under again so soon, or not until they had done a lot more testing, after such a severe reaction but because my cancer was so aggressive, they could only give my body a week to recover. They told me I would have to go back into surgery in seven days and that I could have another reaction, but it was extremely rare. They also decided to take just the one breast because they wanted me to have minimal surgery time.'

Reassured in the days preceding this second surgery by regular contact with her anaesthetist, 'He was amazing. He called me every few days during this time and kept me updated on what was happening, what was going to happen, the risks they were considering. Thinking back on it now, I would like to find him again and say thank you, because he made me feel really calm, and this operation was successful.'

'Would you ever go back to remove the other breast?'

'They are really reluctant to do this. I've been told that for my type of cancer, it's not usually the other breast that it returns in, but rather, somewhere else in the body. So, weighing up the risks versus the benefit, they don't advise it.'

'Going back to your immunotherapy. Had you reached the $60,000? Why did you have to stop?'

'I hadn't quite. With immunotherapy, it works by stimulating your immune system. Kind of puts it into overdrive. This may have been why I had such a severe reaction to the rocuronium. My immune system may have started attacking itself, so it was agreed that it would be better to stop. I had also got the pathology back from my mastectomy which showed that I had had a complete response, that no cancer was detected.'

'No cancer was detected at all in the breast tissue,' I question. 'No evidence of disease?'

'Yes.'

'That's really interesting. It's the benefit of having neo-adjuvant therapy. You can see that the chemotherapy worked. I had chemotherapy second. I don't have that reassurance that it has disappeared.'

'Mine's a good result but it's funny. I don't really think that it does provide any reassurance. It's something that always lingers in my mind. Always. Only time will tell.'

'After all you have gone through, is there anything you think you have learnt from all this?'

'Yes, 100%. It's made a lot of things clearer. Stripped out of life, the things that were meaningless. It's highlighted how important the simple things are in life, like friendships, families, spending time with the people you love. To not take your future for granted. It's also made some of my friendships stronger. Some friends surprised me, friends who I thought would be there for me haven't been and on the flip side, others have stepped up and have been a great support.'

'I agree. I've looked on it as a good time to cull out the friendships you don't want to spend the energy on. I've realised who I want to spend my energy on these days.'

'Exactly. This time has been like a filter.'

'So, you had your operation back in September 2022. And afterwards?'

'That was the end, no further treatment, which I found really hard. I had spent all year wishing for treatment to finish and then when it does, it's very confronting. I felt a bit lost. It was like, ok, you've finished so now get back into the real world, get back to work.'

'Did you work at all during this time?'

'I did. I work from home for Services NSW, and I was really fortunate that they allowed me to arrange my job around treatment. If I needed time off or a lesser workload, then I could organise this. I'm our main income earner and we had not long before my diagnosis bought a house, so it was really fortunate that I could do this. I'm not sure what would have happened otherwise. We probably would have had to sell our home. I'm back working four days a week now.'

'You were fortunate.'

'It's been good in a way, and I've enjoyed the social interaction, but after going through something like breast cancer, sometimes I think I should be going out and doing the bucket list sort of stuff. But the reality is that we are a young family with a mortgage. Things are quite tough at the moment, so packing up and traveling is just not an option.'

'I've spoken with others about people in your situation, your stage of life. We don't know how you do it. Mothers fighting breast cancer, trying to make ends meet. Society is not geared up towards you at all.'

'It's tough. We are doing what we can to adjust, and it may not look how I imagined it, like going around Australia with a caravan, but we are getting away for weekends and such.'

'That leads to my next question. Lifestyle changes. Have you made any?'

'Yes. I'm trying to eat a lot cleaner now. Lots of juicing, green juices, very little meat, and things like that. Exercise has been a struggle. I still haven't gotten my energy back after treatment. It's damaged my heart. I also meditate now and work on reducing my stress.'

'How about supplements?'

'Yes. I see a naturopath who monitors my blood work, my inflammation, my immune system. I've also read Jane McLelland's book and follow a lot of her protocols. I take berberine and curcumin. I'm also on CBD and THC. I use the CBD for inflammation and THC to prevent reoccurrence.'

'To finish, I just have a few more questions. Is there anything you would want someone newly diagnosed to know?'

'Don't be afraid to ask lots of questions. Understand the why behind your treatment. Do your own research. Also, don't just follow the traditional method. Incorporate a holistic approach as well. I'm sure that's why I had such a good response, why I'm NED (no evidence of disease) now, because I was doing all those extra things like juicing and healthy eating. Also, maybe be careful about who you reach out to initially. I found it quite triggering. In the beginning, I found others also going through this and I actually made friends with another young person going through triple negative cancer, but she died three months into her treatment. So be careful.'

'And is there anything you would like someone without cancer to know?'

'I found that after treatment was actually the hardest part, but it's the time when you get the least support. Support comes at the beginning and people think that once you have finished treatment that you are good now, but this was the time I was processing everything and the time that I needed the most emotional support, but it wasn't there.'

When I initially approached people asking if they would be interested in meeting with me for this book, Nicki was the only one who asked why was I doing this? What questions would I ask? Knowing this, I had gone into our interview a little more wary than usual. I hadn't known how it was going to go. How it went was incredibly well, beyond all my expectations. I met a beautiful warrior, kind and generous, who has had to endure and is still enduring hardships no 36-year-old should have to endure. A kind, thoughtful lady with a core of steel and a mesmerising story. After all, there are few out there who can say they died on the operating table.

Addendum

Tricks for coping with your diagnosis - Learn everything you can about your disease. Talk about it. Accept help. Share your experiences. Avail yourself to support organisations and resources.

CHAPTER

33

Michelle-DCIS Hormone Positive

———∿———

MICHELLE'S STORY IS THE LAST I collect and fittingly, it's somewhat different from the others. Creator of the *Little Red Socks, Facebook* page, a page I have mentioned frequently throughout this book, Michelle is someone I have known for years, an old high school friend. I meet with Michelle one Wednesday morning at a popular Byron Bay venue, The Farm. Expecting to share the beautiful open-air property with only a handful of others this mid-week morning, instead we find it teaming with families. We have forgotten that it is the Queensland school holidays. Irrespective, we find a nice place to sit and with chickens clucking at our feet, coffee clutched in our hand, we get down to business. First order of events is a catch-up. We haven't seen each other since my cancer diagnosis and so we spend the first twenty minutes chatting about families, husbands and housing. When we have finished with that, I pull out my notepad and start with my usual questions. What comes is an interesting story heavily entwined with Joy's (Michelle's mother) breast cancer journey. Joy spent 16 years fighting lobular breast cancer the traditional way before succumbing to the disease shortly before Michelle's own diagnosis. Joy's journey heavily influenced Michelle's treatment decisions and many of my questions are answered from both Michelle and Joy's perspective. It makes Michelle's story a little more difficult than others to unravel, but because it is so different, it is certainly worth it.

Unlike others with whom I have met, Michelle doesn't feel a lump, hasn't swollen lymph nodes, doesn't notice an obvious breast change, instead she relies on her intuition that something is wrong. Her intuition has mainly been gained through watching her mother's awful and unsuccessful battle with breast cancer, but it is also based on an acute awareness of her own body. She feels it started about 15 years ago.

Back in around 2007-2008, Michelle suffered a miscarriage. It occurred around the time her not long wed husband was recuperating in hospital following unsuccessful open-heart surgery and at the same time, her mother necessitated a little support. Along with providing this support, Michelle was learning how to be a stepmother to three elder children, mothering her own 18-month-old toddler and, due to her husband's ill health, was the household's primary income earner.

'We had not long been married when Mark had to travel to Sydney for surgery. It failed and he ended up spending 3-4 months down there recovering. At one stage, I didn't know whether he was going to live. Because we had not long been married, our accounts were in separate names. I wasn't able to access money, couldn't pay bills, was finding it hard to pay the mortgage. It was a hugely stressful period and I ended up miscarrying.'

More years pass and if anything, the stress in Michelle's life increases.

'Mum's cancer returned, and the doctors just weren't there for her. The decisions she had to make were terrible. She got radiation poisoning. Her oesophagus failed, and she needed a feeding tube. They kept feeding her with this disgusting formula she hated. When I started blending up nutritious meals and feeding them to her, they switched her tube to a smaller one, making this impossible. She died of starvation in the end. I was also taking on too much work (Michelle is a marriage celebrant), trying to do everything, be everywhere.'

Something has to give and at the age of 45, Michelle suffers another miscarriage.

'This time though, my breasts swelled and when they went down, although they looked the same, something felt different, weird. I just knew something wasn't right.'

Because of her mother's history, Michelle insists on seeing a breast and endocrine specialist, coincidentally Dr Leong, my surgeon, and while nothing shows up in her scans, Michelle continues to remain under Dr Leong's care.

'I felt I needed to keep seeing her. And I had been seeing her for about five or six years, when one of my scans picked something up.'

What Michelle's scan has revealed is ductal carcinoma in situ, a non-invasive cancer contained within the breast tissue. It is hormone positive, HER2 negative.

'Having seen what my mother went through, I wanted a total mastectomy, but Dr Leong recommended a lumpectomy at this stage.'

Michelle undergoes this lumpectomy and surprisingly, the pathology comes back with unclear margins, meaning they may not have removed all of her cancer.

'Another lumpectomy was recommended, but this time I insisted on a double mastectomy. I didn't want the fear of this occurring again. Dr Leong reluctantly agreed, but only if I saw a psychologist first.'

Knowing it's the only way she is going to get her double mastectomy, Michelle meets with a psychologist.

'So I had my operation, and they found another 4.5 cm of tumour hiding behind the nipple. If I hadn't insisted on a mastectomy, then this would have been missed.'

'What did they recommend for treatment?'

'Unlike the private sector where you get to see an oncologist almost immediately, I was public and had to wait six weeks. When I did eventually meet with him, he recommended four chemo sessions and radiation, but I had used these six weeks to do my own research. I saw what the traditional path of chemotherapy and radiation did to my mother. I was sure there had to be alternative options and so I went looking for them.'

As Michelle divulges what she did during this period and afterwards, in her search for answers and fight against breast cancer, I can't help but be impressed. It's obvious that a lot of time, study, money and effort has been required and a lot of tough courageous decisions, made.

'I have a friend who is a highly knowledgeable naturopath. She's also married to an integrative doctor. Straight away, she put me onto Chris Beat Cancer. I also flew to Sydney to meet with her husband and underwent a whole lot of testing with him. I listened to the *Truth about Cancer* podcast along with many other podcasts, read loads of books and did colonics which was really interesting. I did this colonic five weeks after my operation and the blue dye they use to detect your sentinel node was still coming out. This was five weeks later. Imagine how long chemotherapy drugs would last in your system. And I also met Manuela, who I still see today and who has been more helpful than any of my doctors.'

'So at the end of the six weeks, when you got to meet with your oncologist, what did you decide to do? The traditional or the alternative?'

'Despite all my research I was still considering the traditional route, chemotherapy, but before I started, I organised to have an oncotype dx test (a gene profiling test that predicts the likelihood of your cancer returning or your cancer's likely response to treatment). It cost me $6500, and it needed to go to the USA for analysis. Anyway, the result came back that I didn't need to have chemotherapy so although my oncologist was still pushing I have it, I decided not to. He also advised I should take tamoxifen, but after talking with Manuela, I again decided not to follow this advice.'

'How did Manuela help?'

'Initially, Manuela put me on a six-week treatment program. This included a keto diet, Vitamin C infusions two or three times a week, hypobaric oxygen therapy (breathing pure oxygen in a pressurised environment) for one hour some mornings followed by hypothermia treatment (heating the body) to sweat out the toxins in the afternoon. Later, we discussed whether I should take tamoxifen. She advised I could achieve the same result using natural supplements, which is what I decided to do. Each year I also take the Dutch Test, which tests my hormones to monitor that what I am doing is working.'

'And after the six-week program?'

'I continued taking supplements. I didn't stay completely keto, but I looked at my diet, started eating really healthily. Over the following years, I also watched probably in excess of 1000 podcasts. I also found a local health lodge, the Byron Health Lodge, who along with Manuela monitors my pathology and organised for me to take the Greek Cancer test, which can detect even the smallest amount of cancer.'

It was a brave decision to go against an oncologist's advice and it cannot have been an easy one to make, but as she continued on this path, continued successfully following what she calls 'her team's' advice, Michelle knew her decisions were the right ones. Her cancer battle had so far been completely different, so much better, than her mother's. It's a straightforward decision, therefore, in late 2019, following a diagnosis of parathyroid adenoma (a benign tumour of the parathyroid gland), to add another integrative medical specialist to her support group, a practitioner of Chinese medicine.

'If I could go back and choose what I wanted to do again, then I would choose to study Chinese medicine.' Michelle tells me. 'It has been amazing. My doctor immediately identified that the cold juices and salads I was eating were wrong for me and changed me to a warm food diet. Two weeks later and my thyroid problems were gone. I still have the tumour, which is due to be removed next month, but all the other problems associated with it like the lump in my throat, went.'

'So, five years down the track, where are you up to with everything?'

'In 2021, I was dismissed by my oncologist two years early. He said that obviously what I was doing was working, and that there was no longer any need for me to see him. I still see Dr Leong each year and have an annual ultrasound. I still take my supplements, am still working with Manuela, my Chinese doctor, the Byron Health lodge and also, a nearby wellness centre.'

'That leads me on to one of my generic questions. Have you made any lifestyle changes since your diagnosis?' We both laugh at my question. It's pretty obvious that Michelle has made many life changes since her diagnosis. She gives me an answer, however.

'One of the first things we did was install water filters throughout our entire house, so now I drink, wash and bathe, in filtered water. I'm very aware of environmental toxins, so only use natural makeups, perfumes, shampoos, soaps, laundry powders. One day I just gathered everything up and gave it all away to my friends. I bought an infrared sauna to detox. I drink much less alcohol now. While we eat some meat, our diet is mainly plant based. I do Pilates two or three times per week for bone strength. I walk to the Byron Lighthouse regularly. I have learnt to meditate. The best thing, though, is that I have educated my daughter about all of this. She was only 12 when I had my mastectomy and knowing her grandmother had also had breast cancer, she had asked me if she was going to be next. I had replied that I was going to do everything I could to prevent that from happening. She was a huge reason for all of my changes. I am determined that she won't go through what mum and I have been through.'

'Our kids are definitely the best reason for change,' I agree. 'So, you've mentioned alternative therapies and environmental toxins. Is there anything else that really comes to the fore regarding what you have learnt on this journey?'

'To be kind to yourself. For years, work came first. I pushed family and friends aside. Now I know what's important. I've also learnt that kindness goes a long way, to treat others how I would like to be treated.

You can still get your point across, still achieve what you want, but be kind doing so, don't be judgemental. Also cost. A lot of my treatments have been expensive, but my life and my family are worth it.'

'And for someone newly diagnosed with breast cancer, is there anything you would like them to know?'

Michelle is quick and adamant with her response.

'When you are first diagnosed, don't rush into anything, don't get pushed into decisions. You have time to think about what you would like to do. Your cancer has, more than likely, been growing for years. It will not change in the next two or so weeks, so take time to process everything. Without that six-week gap while waiting to see an oncologist, I may have taken a completely different path. I had a friend, Ros, who was diagnosed at the exact time I was, with triple negative breast cancer. I watched as she was pushed into chemotherapy and all sorts of decisions. It turned out that she was BRCA positive (a harmful gene highly associated with an increased risk of breast cancer), but they didn't find this out until later. It may have changed her initial treatment. I watched as she got worse and worse, yet kept following what they told her until she died. She was never in control of her own illness. So, be the master of your treatment.'

'And for those without breast cancer. Anything you could tell them?'

'Manage your stress levels. Stress played a large part in my cancer diagnosis. Learn to meditate. Do something nice for yourself. Even if it's as simple as going for a walk or having a nice bath, just do it. Women don't look after themselves enough. We take too much on, so I would tell them or anyone, to look after yourself, to prioritise yourself.'

It was always going to be interesting meeting with Michelle. She had been the first in my high school cohort (that I knew of), who had been diagnosed with a life-threatening illness; thus she was someone I had been concerned about and taken an interest in. So much so that I had been a regular follower of her *Facebook* page, even before my own diagnosis. I had been keen to meet with her, keen to hear firsthand, her journey. Now that I have done so, I leave feeling quite in awe of what she has learnt, implemented and achieved. To refuse chemotherapy and hormone therapy is no light decision, but Michelle has done this, following her own gut feeling. She has replaced them with natural alternatives following hundreds of hours of study, incredible dedication to her cause, and the accumulation of a great support team. That her oncologist dismissed her two years early is proof that what she has been doing has been successful. Walking away from our meeting, I can't help wondering what I would have done in her situation. Somehow, I don't think I would have been as brave.

Addendum

After active treatment – Unless you have been diagnosed metastatic and will stay in active treatment for the rest of your life, you will next transition to follow-up care. Unfortunately, this may feel inadequate, even non-existent, so learn to be your own advocate. Follow up all niggles. Look after yourself.

CHAPTER
34

Epilogue

———————

IT'S THE END OF JUNE now, 18 months since I was told I had breast cancer. Active treatment is far behind me. Those long tough months overshadowed by Covid are, but a strange memory, and I have finished meeting with my fellow fighters, finished obtaining their remarkable stories. There is not much more to say, which means it's time to wrap this story up, to put it to bed. It's not been the easiest book to write. An aftereffect of chemotherapy is brain fog, but somewhere within this annoying cloud that fills my head, I have found a tale, a book that's been both enjoyable and cathartic to write. More so when, tucked within a café somewhere, I would hear the journey of fellow survivors. It was always an incredible experience when I met up with these ladies. In the majority of cases, I would have no inkling beforehand of what I was about to hear, no idea at all about their journeys. Many is the time I would finish an interview feeling absolutely dumbfounded from what

I had been told, what I had learnt. To hear Oxana talk about her initial misdiagnosis and to hear how she blames the thoughts in her head for her cancer reoccurrence was educational, as was comparing the stories of Justine and Julie. I met with Julie a week after meeting with Justine and never could two tales be so different. Julie, 20 years a cancer survivor who, following her diagnosis, never stopped drinking nor smoking and Justine, someone who completely changed all aspects of her life. A keto following, ultra-healthy, toxicity free, warrior. From these two, I've learnt that as everyone's cancer diagnosis is different, so too is the way they approach it, their treatment, and the end response.

It was lovely meeting beautiful, courageous Polly and her cheeky little miracle daughter, Ayla. Conceiving naturally after such heavy chemo, Polly is living proof of just how incredible, how tough the female body can be. And it was quite poignant meeting with feisty Bianca, at 25, the youngest breast cancer warrior I have met. It felt so unfair that someone so young should be going through this. She should have been out there discovering life, moving forward, not putting it on hold to fight what is supposed to be an older person's disease. And gorgeous Nicki who died on the operating table but lived to tell the tale. One of only two ladies I met who managed to keep working during their treatment, she also had to continue in her role as mother to four, mostly young, children. I'm in awe of her. Michelle's story was also an eye-opener, the only person I know who has successfully eschewed traditional treatment. An incredibly brave lady who went in search of her own answers.

And myself, a few months onwards, where am I at? First, I'm seeing Doc Martin trimonthly now, to be followed by six then 12-monthly appointments for the next eight years as he monitors my blood levels and the mass in my chest. It's a bit of a mixed blessing really, this mass. Disconcertingly, when active treatment for breast cancer is finished, that's it. Current medical policy advocates no immediate follow-up scans. No ultrasound. No MRI. Cancer marker blood tests (blood tests that search for substances made by cancer or abnormal cells), are not recommended by mainstream practitioners. You're deemed cured for now, and unless you feel a pain somewhere or something crops up, that's it. At least by having my chest mass scanned regularly, I have some reassurance that my cancer hasn't returned (or at least, not in this area of my body). Others don't have this comfort. And an immense comfort it is. I cannot stress how much breast cancer survivors live in fear that their cancer will return.

Dr Martin is also monitoring the effects of the letrozole and abemaciclib. Unfortunately, the main side-effects of these still haven't changed. Letrozole causes terrible muscle and joint pain. I often refer to myself as a wizened old lady the way letrozole makes my body feel and move. Like Karen, one lady whom I interviewed, I also suspect that this drug is toying with my head. I no longer seem to feel the great exciting highs or the deep anxious lows caused by what life throws at you. I just seem to exist on an anesthetised, detached plane now. For example, whereas once I used to get butterflies of excitement when organising future travel or after a good bowls win, now I feel a little indifferent, slightly numb. I am certainly not the happy-go-lucky, carefree person I used to be, and I miss that person.

That was letrozole, with the abemaciclib, it's lethargy and nausea. I am 9 months in now with 15 more to go, and I am still finding it difficult to exercise. Still getting incredibly fatigued. Long gone are the days that I could reach 10,000 daily steps. Fortunately, I've avoided one of those really horrendous diarrhoea episodes experienced by others on this drug, although I do suffer with it frequently, mainly in the mornings.

At one of my earlier post treatment visits, Doc Martin convinced me to purchase Prolia. 'It can give you an extra 1% chance of avoiding cancer reoccurrence in the bones', so, still determined to do everything I can to beat this, each six months I give myself an injection.

My eyesight is still causing a few problems. It doesn't appear to be worsening, but equally, it's not getting any better. I'm due to see Dr Stephenson again shortly. Fingers crossed, she'll just tell me to come back next year. A response I also hope to get from Dr Leong when I met with her again in August for my 12-monthly check-up.

Physically, I still weigh 53 kilos, and I still look bony. My new diet of mainly plant-based food with very little dairy means my weight and physique probably won't change much or at least not while I am taking my nausea producing, appetite suppressing, diarrhoea generating, medication. I'm still consuming supplements, still drinking green tea, still having regular lymphatic drainage massages, still avoiding alcohol, except on very special occasions, and still wearing my hair short. My chest scars have healed incredibly well. I have embraced my flat chest, thrown away every bra I owned and my prostheses are growing cobwebs at the bottom of a deep, dark drawer. Although challenging, I know it's helping, so I am still doing my yoga stretches daily and I still sometimes need to spend a good part of the day on the couch. A good night's sleep is still a forgotten luxury despite finally being able to sleep on my side again, with discomfort and exhausting hot flashes still wakening me numerous times a night. Darryl and I still live half the week at Brunswick Heads, the other half at Coolangatta, and still go for our ritual morning coffee.

Last week, I met with Dr Binjemain again. Being an integrative practitioner, he supports cancer marker blood tests and so is monitoring my CA 15-3 and CA 27.29 levels. I am unsure if this is a worthwhile exercise; the jury is still out on these tests, but again I'll reiterate, I am going to do everything I can to beat this breast cancer. He also educated me on the toxic effects of mould, important in our region where high humidity and high rainfall are common.

'Exposure to mould can increase aromatase activity (the conversion of hormones to estrogen) by up to 339% and increase oestradiol (the most potent form of estrogen) levels by up to 300%. Something you, with a hormone driven cancer, need to avoid.'

I also learnt that maybe my cancer is more glutamine than glucose driven.

'Your cancer didn't show up in your original PET scan,' he had stated after reading the relevant report. 'PET scans use glucose to highlight cancerous areas. The fact that nothing showed up would indicate that your tumours were not feeding on glucose, but something else such as glutamine.' Not all that familiar with glutamine, I leave his office with some homework to do.

After going through an extensive training program, last Saturday, I commenced my first shift as a Gold Coast Airport Ambassador. This shift coincided with not only the first day of the New South Wales school holidays, but with some pretty wild weather. It meant many flights were cancelled, many travellers were left stranded, and I was certainly kept busy appeasing and redirecting passengers. Needless to say, I loved it.

Finally, I find it only fair to ask myself those three questions I asked my fellow fighters. Namely, what has this journey taught me? Is there anything I could share with someone newly diagnosed and do I have anything to say to those without cancer?

First, reading back over what I have written and I realise that this breast cancer adventure has taught me a great deal. Foremost is to live my life. Odds are, my cancer could return at any moment, so do what I can and want, now. Go for my daily coffee, organise my next holiday, join more classes at the University of the 3rd Age, get a breast cancer tattoo on my right wrist, join a second bowling club, purchase some funky glasses to go with my new short hair. And appreciate the mundane—the green trees, the blue ocean, the birds singing, that comfortable accommodating couch.

I have also learnt not to fear death. I've accepted that it may happen to me sooner than I expected, so I'm not going to sweat over it. As they say, it happens to everyone. In this same vein, I've learnt to appreciate growing older, blowing out another candle. Age is a privilege.

I always thought Darryl, after his horrendous accident that left him with so many ailments, would die before me. Now, I don't know, so, I've learnt not to make life assumptions.

Having breast cancer has also taught me the true value of family and friends. I could not have endured this journey without Darryl's unwavering support. My mum, step-mum, sister- and sister-in-law's food packages. Paige's exciting parcels and thoughtful advice. Pierce's upbeat weekly check-ins. My bowling buddies' friendship. They say the worst of times can bring out the best in people and in my situation, I found this true.

On the other hand, I have also lost allies, personally experienced the meaning of fair-weathered friends. The ones I haven't heard nor seen since my diagnosis. I'm not letting it worry me; instead I've now learnt that I don't have to waste valuable energy on those who can't reciprocate it.

Second, do I have any advice for those newly diagnosed? While I wholeheartedly agree with every answer given by all those I interviewed for this book, what's had the biggest impact on my life, and what I advocate more than anything, is the importance of a healthy lifestyle. To limit foods containing hormones. Reduce or cut out entirely, meat, sugar and dairy. Exercise daily. Pay attention to environmental and behavioural toxicities. Take regular supplements. While I understand my choices are not the answer for everyone, I know they are working for me. Cancer was obviously my wake-up call for change. Currently, I am looking the best I have for years and whereas once debilitating headaches were a frequent event, occurring two or three times per week, since introducing these lifestyle amendments, I have had just a few.

And finally, to those without cancer, is there anything I have to say to you? Well, yes, a couple of things. Firstly, are you at risk? Do you over-consume? Do you have any current trigger warnings like my dimple, Karen's sore back, Nicki's swollen lymph node, Oxana's swelling boobs? If the answer to any of these is yes, then do something about it. Don't leave it too long. Don't become a stage 4 when you could be a stage 0.

And secondly, is what most of those interviewed have said. It's to not be afraid to talk to someone with cancer about their diagnosis. Ask them questions. Listen to their answers. Learn from them. Offer support if need be. Don't make the subject about you. Don't treat them any differently. I can't tell you the number of times I have told someone that I spent most of 2022 fighting breast cancer only to have them not say a single word in response. Either they go mute, or, they change the subject. I mentioned earlier having lunch with two close friends and neither of them made any mention at all to my cancer. The opportunity never arose for me to bring the subject up myself, so a major part of my new identity was just ignored. I'm still trying to fathom why. Why are people so scared to talk about cancer with someone who has cancer and is this you?

It's funny, I ended my last book reminding people of the idiom Carpe diem, 'seize the day'. Given what has happened since I wrote those words, never was a reminder so appropriate, so prophetic, so I'll finish this book with another pertinent phrase, a quote attributed to Abraham Lincoln. A missive I find particularly relevant following my breast cancer diagnosis.

'In the end, it's not the years in your life that count. It's the life in your years.'

GLOSSARY

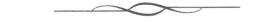

Abemaciclib: A medication that targets cancer cells and stops them growing and dividing.

Acupuncture: A Chinese medicine that uses fine needles to penetrate the skin.

Adjuvant therapy: Chemotherapy after surgery.

Anaesthetist: A specialist doctor responsible for providing anaesthesia to patients.

Angiosarcoma: A rare soft tissue tumour of the breast

Antihistamine: A medication that helps with allergies.

Arimidex: An aromatase inhibitor.

Aromatase activity: The conversion of hormones to estrogen.

Aromatase inhibitor: A type of hormone drug used to treat breast cancer and given to women who have gone through natural menopause.

Axillary lymph node dissection: Surgery to remove lymph nodes.

Bisphosphonates: The use of drugs to block various causes of cancer growth.

BRCA positive: A harmful gene highly associated with an increased risk of breast cancer.

Breast biopsy: A procedure to remove a sample of breast tissue for testing.

Breast prosthesis: An artificial breast.

Breast reconstruction: Surgery to recreate a breast.

CA 15-3 and CA 27.29 tests: Blood tests to monitor response to breast cancer treatment.

Cancer marker blood tests: Blood tests that search for substances made by cancer or abnormal cells.

Cannula: A thin tube inserted into a vein to administer medication.

CBC: Complete blood count.

CBD: A chemical found in marijuana.

Chemo induced neuropathy: Nerve damage that can cause lifelong numbness or tingling in your hands, fingers, toes and feet.

Chemotherapy: The use of powerful chemicals to kill cancer cells.

Chiropractor: A health care professional specialising in diagnosing and treating musculoskeletal issues through spinal adjustments.

Chronic obstructive pulmonary disease or COPD: A common lung disease.

Coffee enemas: The cleansing of your rectum by using coffee.

Compression stockings or TEDS: Compression garments to support circulation.

Cording: Cord-like structures that run from your armpit under the skin on your inner-arm and also known as axillary web syndrome.

Core needle biopsy: The use of a hollow needle to obtain a sample of breast tissue.

CT scan: A series of x-rays that reveals a 3D image of your body.

DCIS: Abnormal cells inside a breast milk duct.

Deep inspiration breath hold or DIBH: A breathing technique to reduce radiation dosage to your heart.

DIEP reconstruction: Reconstructing a breast using the body's fat, skin and blood vessels.

Doxorubicin: A chemotherapy drug used to treat cancer.

Dry brushing: Brushing the skin to stimulate the lymphatic system.

Ductal carcinoma in situ: Abnormal cells inside a breast milk duct.

Dutch Test: A blood test which will provide an analysis of your hormones.

Ectopic heartbeat: Where your heart beats too fast.

Electrocardiogram: A test to record the electrical activity of your heart.

Endocrine: Relates to glands which secrete hormones or other products directly into the blood.

Extra-nodal extension: Where the tumour has perforated the lymph node capsule.

Fibroadenomas: Solid, smooth benign lumps.

Fibromyalgia: Widespread pain throughout your whole body.

Flap reconstruction: Reconstructing a breast using the bodies fat, skin and blood vessels.

Grade: How abnormal a cancer cell appears under a microscope compared to a normal cell.

Greek Cancer test: A blood test which will isolate and identify cancer cells.

Gynaecologist: A doctor specialising in the female reproductive system.

Heparin: A blood thinner

HER2 positive breast cancer: A cancer with too much of a protein called Human Epidermal growth factor Receptor 2 on their surface compared to normal cells.

Herceptin: A cancer drug that targets HER2 positive cancers.

Hormone blockers: Drugs used to treat hormone positive cancers.

Hormone receptor-positive breast cancer: Cancers that need the female hormones oestrogen and/or progesterone to grow and reproduce.

Hormone Replacement Therapy or HRT: Replacing hormones to treat the effects of menopause.

Hot flushes: A sudden feeling of warmth throughout the body.

Hypobaric oxygen therapy: Breathing pure oxygen in a pressurised environment.

Hypothermia treatment: Heating the body.

Hysterectomy: Removal of a woman's uterus.

Immunologist: A doctor who treats immune system problems.

Immunotherapy: Uses substances either made in a laboratory or by the body to help the immune system do a better job.

Implant reconstruction: Reconstructing a breast using implants.

Inflammatory breast cancer: A rare type of cancer that makes a breast red and swollen; this cancer can occur in either the ducts or lobes and tends to spread faster than the other types.

Infra-red saunas: The use of infrared heaters to warm the body.

Invasive ductal carcinoma: Cancer formed in the milk duct that has spread into the surrounding breast tissue.

Invasive lobular carcinoma: Cancer formed in the milk lobe that has spread into the surrounding breast tissue.

Ketogenic diet: A high fat, medium protein, low carb diet.

Kinase: A protein that helps cells grow and divide.

Letrozole: An aromatase inhibitor used in fighting breast cancer.

Lobular carcinoma in situ or LCIS: The formation of abnormal cells in the milk lobes.

Lumpectomy: Surgery to remove the cancer only and spare the breast.

Lymphatic drainage massage: Gentle manipulation and light skin stretching to promote the movement of lymph fluid around the body.

Lymphoedema: Swelling that occurs when lymph nodes or vessels become blocked.

Mammogram: An x-ray picture of your breast.

Mastectomy: A surgical operation to remove a breast.

Medicare Enhanced Primary Care plan: A plan of management that will enable you to access services such as physiotherapy or occupational therapy.

Meditation: A practice used to induce a clear and calm state.

Melatonin: A hormone produced in the brain that controls the body's day and night cycles.

Meningioma: Benign brain tumours.

Menopause: It is the time that marks the end of a woman's menstrual cycles.

Metastasis: This means when cancer has spread from its original site to another part of the body.

MRI: A non-invasive procedure that uses magnetic fields and radio waves to take a cross examination of your body.

NED: No evidence of disease.

Neo-adjuvant treatment: Chemotherapy before surgery.

Neutropenia sepsis: An infection in those with a low white blood cell count.

Niacin detox: Using niacin, exercise and heat to eliminate toxins from the body.

Oestradiol: The most potent form of estrogen.

Oestrogen: One of the main female sex hormones.

Oncologist: A doctor who treats someone with cancer.

Oncotype dx test: A gene profiling test that predicts the likelihood of your cancer returning or your cancer's likely response to treatment.

Osteoporosis: A condition where bones become weak and brittle.

Paclitaxel: A chemotherapy drug used to treat cancer.

Paget's disease of the Nipple: A rare form of breast cancer that causes breast skin changes.

Papillary carcinoma: A rare form of breast cancer that appears as an irregular solid mass.

Parathyroid adenoma: A benign tumour of the parathyroid gland.

Perimenopause: The transition to menopause.

PET scan: An imaging test that shows how internal body organs and tissue are working.

Phlebotomist: A person who takes blood.

Phyllodes tumours: Smooth, firm lumps in the breast.

Physiotherapist: A qualified health professional expert in the structure and movement of the human body.

Portacath: A device that is planted under the skin on the chest wall to draw blood and give treatment such as chemotherapy drugs or antibiotics.

PPE: Personal protective equipment

Progesterone: A hormone that supports menstruation and maintaining pregnancy.

Prolia: A medication used to prevent or treat osteoporosis.

Psoriatic arthritis: A type of inflammatory arthritis.

Radiation Therapy: The treatment of cancer using x-rays.

Radiation burn: A side-effect of radiation therapy.

Radiographer: A qualified health professional who takes x-rays and other medical images.

Reiki: A Japanese form of therapy to promote well-being.

Ribociclib: A CDK 4/6 inhibitor.

Rocuronium: A muscle relaxant.

Sentinel node biopsy: A procedure to see if cancer has spread.

Seroma: A pool of fluid under the skin.

Sonographer: A health care professional who specialises in using ultrasound.

Stage: How big a cancer is and whether it has spread.

Steroids: Anti-inflammatory medications.

Tamoxifen: Hormone therapy used to treat hormone positive breast cancer.

Tissue expander: An empty breast implant that will be expanded to create a new breast.

Triple Negative breast cancer: Does not have any of the three common receptors found on breast cancer cells (oestrogen, progesterone or HER2).

Ultrasound: The use of sound waves to produce a picture of the inside of the body.

Verzenio: Targeted therapy for the treatment of hormone positive breast cancer.

Warfarin: An anticoagulant used to treat and prevent blood clots.

ACKNOWLEDGMENTS

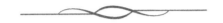

A DIAGNOSIS OF BREAST CANCER changes your life forever. I am never going to be the person I was. I would like to thank the following who stood with me, supported me and provided for me as I transformed from the old Emma into the new. My family—in particular Darryl, mum, Michelle, Paige, Pierce, Patma and Petria. The John Flynn medical staff—in particular Dr Martin and Dr Leong. The amazing fighters, friends and survivors who constitute the Women's Cancer Support GC group—in particular, its founder Sandra. My bowling buddies—The Brunswick Broomstick Riders who always manage to cheer me up.

I would especially like to thank the eleven amazing warriors who allowed me to share their story and without whom, I would not have a book—Tracey, Karen R, Kelly, Oxana, Karen G, Justine, Julie, Polly, Bianca, Nicki and Michelle.

MORE FROM
EMMA SCATTERGOOD

I WRITE MY ADVENTURE BOOKS with two purposes in mind. The first is to share my experiences with you - whether it be an awe-inspiring glimpse of an ancient civilisation at Petra, a thrilling train ride across Mongolia, the feeling of loneliness as you cross the Atlantic Ocean or what it's like having your breasts amputated. I also write for informative reasons. If you can learn something from my books, then I have been successful. Of course, I hope that you can learn many things.

If you have enjoyed reading *My Breast Cancer Adventure*, **please leave a review.**
Where to leave a review -

Amazon - https://www.amazon.com/stores/Emma-Scattergood/author/
Goodreads - https://www.goodreads.com/author/Emma_Scattergood
Bookbub - https://www.bookbub.com/profile/emma-scattergood?list=about

If you would like to know more about me, please visit –
https://linktr.ee/emmascattergood
or browse my website –
http://darmatravels.com

PREVIOUS BOOKS BY EMMA SCATTERGOOD

Bucket Lists & Walking Sticks
A Terrible Accident. Forced Retirement.
An Excuse to Pull Out the Bucket List!

After a motorbike accident leaves her husband with life-changing injuries, author Emma organises a worldwide adventure based on the contents of an old, laminated bucket list.

It will be the journey of a lifetime, seeking health and ticking off list items: from viewing ancient Petra and treading Greece's Parthenon to traversing the Suez Canal and hunting down Doc Martin.

Taking seven months and spanning Asia and Europe, this journal, told in mouth-watering and humorous detail, will pull you headlong into the sights, life, culture and beauty of each place visited. It will make you want to follow in their footsteps.

Itchy Feet and Bucket Lists

I've pulled the Bucket List back out.
Amongst what's left are the Trans-Siberian Express,
the Terracotta Army, the Swiss Alps and the Panama Canal.

Easy words spoken - catalyst for an unforgettable adventure across the steppes of Mongolia, the wilderness of Siberia, Putin's Russia. Through Europe during winter and over the lonely Atlantic and Pacific Oceans.

Commencing in October 2019 and undertaken by author Emma and husband Darryl, the journey will provide lessons on a developing pandemic, Google translate, food poisoning and train accidents. Throw in some goals like having a rum in Barbados, a coffee in Guatemala and guacamole in Mexico; it might even be the cure for their (or your) itchy feet.